Neurohumoral Maintenance
of Immune Homeostasis

NEUROHUMORAL MAINTENANCE
Translated and edited by Samuel A

Elena A. Korneva
Viktor M. Klimenko
Elenora K. Shkhinek

)F IMMUNE HOMEOSTASIS
orson and Elizabeth O'Leary Corson

In collaboration with
Roland Dartau, Justina Epp,
and L. A. Mutschler

The University of Chicago Press
Chicago and London

Elena A. Korneva, Viktor M. Klimenko, and **Elenora K. Shkhinek** are all members of the Institute for Experimental Medicine of the USSR Academy of Medical Sciences in Leningrad.

Samuel A. Corson, emeritus professor at Ohio State University, has been a faculty member in psychiatry, biophysics, Slavic and Eastern European studies, biomedical engineering, and education. **Elizabeth O'Leary Corson** is a research associate in the Department of Psychiatry at the Ohio State University College of Medicine.

This book is a translation of
Neyrogumoral'noye obespecheniye immunnogo gomeostaza
(Leningrad: Nauka Publishers, 1978),
including a new epilogue by Elena A. Korneva

The University of Chicago Press, Chicago 60637
The University of Chicago Press, Ltd., London

Library of Congress Cataloging in Publication Data

Korneva, E. A. (Elena Andreevna)
    Neurohumoral maintenance of immune homeostasis.

    Translation of: Neïrogumoral 'noe obespechenie immunnogo gomeostaza.
    Bibliography: p.
    Includes index.
    1. Immune response—Regulation. 2. Neuroendocrinology.
I. Klimenko, V. M. (Viktor Matveevich) II. Shkhinek,
E. K. (Eleonora Konstantinovna) III. Title. [DNLM:
1. Immunity. 2. Homeostasis. 3. Nervous System—
Physiology. QW 504 K84n]
QR186.K6713   1985   616.07'9   84-8771
ISBN 0-226-45042-2

Contents

	Editors' Preface	vii
	Introduction	1
1	Major Stages in the Investigation of the Influence of the Nervous System on Immune Processes	5
	Elena A. Korneva	
2	The Sympathoadrenal System and Immune Reactions	14
	Elena A. Korneva	
3	The Influence of the Hypothalamus on Immune Reactions	28
	Elena A. Korneva	
4	Neural Hypothalamic Mechanisms in the Development of an Immune Response	55
	Viktor M. Klimenko	
5	Hormones and the Immune Response	98
	Elenora K. Shkhinek	
6	Organization of the System of Neurohumoral Regulation of Immune Homeostasis: Perspectives and Methods of Investigation (General Conclusions)	159
	Epilogue	168
	Elena A. Korneva	
	References	173
	Author Index	239
	Subject Index	249

Editors' Preface

As early as 1883, the distinguished Russian pathologist Il'ya Il'ich Mechnikov presented at a meeting of the Society of Physicians and Scientists in Odessa, Russia, a report on the role of phagocytosis in the defense mechanisms utilized by organisms in combating infectious diseases. This represented a significant contribution to the development of the concept of immunity, for which Mechnikov and Paul Ehrlich eventually were awarded the Nobel prize in 1908.

Mechnikov was a contemporary of the physiologist I. M. Sechenov, the clinician S. P. Botkin, and the physiologist I. P. Pavlov, whose collaboration led to the development of the theory of nervism, or the neurogenic theory in biology and medicine.

The essence of the theory of nervism can be summarized as follows:

1. All living processes, including consciousness, can ultimately be analyzed in terms of natural laws. However, the specific configuration of materials forming living organisms endows them with properties not possessed by the individual components. The properties of H_2O or H_2O_2 do not represent merely a summation of the properties of the component elements. A new quality is represented in a molecule of H_2O or H_2O_2, this quality being determined by the specific configuration of the elements. The appearance of a new quality in a chemical compound does not compel the chemist to resort to mysticism in explaining the properties of water or of a tobacco mosaic virus molecule. By the same reasoning, a biologist need not invoke mystical vitalism to explain the properties of living matter. A biolo-

vii

gist or a chemist could choose to resort to mysticism, but this type of approach fails to provide either understanding, prediction, or control.

2. Nature contains many hierarchies of organization and configuration of matter, each level possessing characteristic qualities. The quality we call "life" appeared at a particular level of organization of certain material entities. Consciousness and mind are qualities characteristic of a certain level of organization of neural elements.

3. Living organisms are characterized by a hierarchy of different levels of integration, beginning with intracellular integration and leading up to integration of organs and organ systems by means of a central nervous system. In higher animals, the central nervous system itself is structured on the basis of integrated hierarchical levels, the cerebral cortex assuming a progressively increasing dominant role in animals higher in the evolutionary scale. Cerebrovisceral theory emphasizes that this increase in cerebral dominance in higher animals also holds for visceral and endocrine functions.

4. The progressively increasing dominance of the cerebral mantle in higher organisms, especially in man, and the resulting increase in the multiplicity of physiological responses to *symbols* of physicochemical stimuli, multiplied the possibilities for psychological factors to impinge on somatic and visceral functions. Consequently, the Sechenov-Botkin-Pavlov neurogenic theory led to an emphasis on the importance of psychosocial factors in diagnosis, therapy, and prophylaxis. Thus was prepared the physiological basis for psychosomatic medicine.

As an illustration of the practical application of the theory of nervism, one may cite the clinical orientation of S. P. Botkin (see Corson 1957). For example, Botkin looked upon fever as a defense mechanism (in which the central nervous system played an important role) and did not encourage the excessive use of drugs to combat fevers, a practice that was fashionable in medical circles at that time. He advocated using drugs with care and only when definitely indicated. Botkin suggested the need for studying the mechanisms the organism used in combating disease: "It is in this studying of the natural abortive forms (of disease), the learning of the methods used by the organism in combating infection, it appears to me, that we

shall find that path that will lead us to the discovery of recuperating, disease-combating remedies" (see also Corson and Corson 1975).

Mechnikov and Sechenov maintained a close friendship for many years. The theory of nervism played a major role in Mechnikov's overall biomedical orientation and in the development of the idea of immunity as a major factor in health maintenance.

It is thus natural that the theory of nervism and that of immunology eventually gave rise to the concept of neuroimmunology, and that Russian biomedical scientists have played a pioneering role in developing experimental studies in this area. This book by Elena A. Korneva and her colleagues summarizes some of these studies conducted in the USSR and in the West. This exciting area of research has also been referred to as "neuroimmunomodulation" (Spector 1981) and as "psychoneuroimmunology" (Ader 1981).

The authors review the following types of studies (chiefly from Soviet laboratories):

1. Pavlovian conditioning studies on immune responses. A critical review is presented of experiments purporting to demonstrate Pavlovian conditional immune responses as well as of studies reporting negative results.

2. Studies on the effects of ablation and stimulation of various hypothalamic structures on immune responses.

3. Effects of endogenous and exogenous hormones on immune reactions, with particular reference to hormones of the hypothalamohypophysio-adrenal system.

4. Studies on neurophysiological changes in the central nervous system (particularly in the posterior hypothalamic areas and in the amygdala) associated with primary and secondary immune reactions.

Introduction

Immune homeostasis as a concept is currently being widely used, though not always correctly. This term is usually used to define a complex of processes in the organism that ensure the constancy of genetically predetermined cellular characteristics. At the highest stages of evolution, the immune system carries out this function; that is, strictly speaking, we are dealing with homeostasis supported by immunologic means. In essence, this represents an organismic approach to living systems.

Whereas at the early stages of development of immunology it was believed that these mechanisms primarily give protection against infections, it has now become apparent how extensive the functions of the immune system are in maintaining genetic constancy of the cellular makeup of the organism in general. According to Bernett (1971), Petrov (1976), and Kaznacheyev and Subbotin (1971), this includes the destruction of mutant cells that differ genetically from the forms characteristic of a given organism.

The trigger for immune reactions is the action of an antigen, that is, a genetically foreign substance, while the final stage of these reactions is the formation of defense factors, that is, cellular or humoral antibodies specific to a given antigen. In regard to its onset and completion, the process is specific. However, nonspecific reactions (which in the integrated organism are intimately linked with specific resistance mechanisms) play a substantial part in its implementation. This relationship is determined by at least three basic factors.

1. Under natural conditions, antigens as a rule enter the organism not in the form of chemically pure protein, but as complexes with

1

other substances, which leads to nonspecific reactions of various kinds: inflammation, fever, the stimulation of various chemoreceptors, and so on. Pure antigen can have the same effects.

2. The development of the immune response includes nonspecific phases, for example, the macrophage reaction.

3. Hormonal and neural influences are of substantial importance in ensuring an immune reaction of adequate intensity.

Neurohumoral factors that have a regulatory role in the maintenance of immune homeostasis can be considered nonspecific components of specific immune processes. Whereas the qualitative nature of the immune response is determined by the properties of the antigen, its intensity is determined not only by the nature and amount of the antigen, but also by a number of other factors, including neurohumoral agents.

The methods of studying the neurohumoral maintenance of immune homeostasis do not differ in principle from those used to study the regulation of any other function. They comprise a physiological analysis of the paths taken by the influx into the nervous system of information about the entry of antigen into the organism and an examination of the central components of the regulatory system and of the means of transmitting efferent messages to the effector organs.

However, the peculiarities of the structure and function of the immune system necessitate a search for special approaches and methods permitting us to apply accepted or modified procedures of neurophysiologic analysis to specific aspects of the problem under study. For example, studying the neurophysiological correlates of immunogenesis required, because of the long-term and multicomponent nature of this process, the development of a special mathematical procedure for analyzing data on the impulse activity of individual cerebral neurons.

In recent years there has been a considerable increase in interest in the neurohumoral regulation of immune homeostasis. This is evidenced not only by the publication of monographs (Kozlov 1973; Frolov 1974; Kesztyüs 1967), but also by the organization of two all-Union symposia on this problem. These studies have constituted a dialogue among immunologists, physiologists, and morphologists, thus permitting the investigation of this problem at different levels of organization from the cellular to the organismic.

A number of pressing clinical problems indicate the need to influence the intensity of immune processes; for example, the widespread use of tissue and organ transplantation and the investigation of the nature and treatment of allergic and autoimmune components in the pathogenesis of many diseases.

Among possible ways of influencing the course of immune processes, it is rational to utilize those that exist in the body and are capable of regulating the intensity of immune reactions and of maintaining the constancy of the protein composition of the organism under changing environmental conditions. The search for influences of this kind requires an understanding of the neural, endocrine, and other humoral mechanisms of regulation of immune homeostasis. The results of such investigations are presented in this book.

At the present level of understanding, this problem is still far from being solved, and the available data should be regarded as first steps on a long and difficult road. Nevertheless, the physiological analysis of individual components of the process of regulation of immune reactions presented here, together with data in the literature, makes it possible even now to propose a concept of a system of neurohumoral maintenance of immune homeostasis and, on the basis of this working hypothesis, to suggest methods for further study.

The work on this problem at the Institute of Experimental Medicine of the USSR Academy of Medical Sciences was initiated by academicians D. A. Biryukov and V. I. Ioffe (USSR Academy of Medical Sciences). The immunologic part of most of the experiments described in chapters 2 and 3 was carried out at the Section of Microbiology and Immunology of the Institute of Experimental Medicine of the USSR Academy of Medical Sciences by candidate of medical sciences L. M. Khay under the direction of V. I. Ioffe. The morphological studies of the brain were performed by candidates of biological sciences M. V. Medvedeva and I. P. Tsvetkova, and the computer processing of the electrophysiological data was done at the laboratory headed by Doctor of Medical Sciences N. I. Moiseyeva. Part of the research on the participation of hormones of the hypophyseoadrenal system in reactions to antigens was conducted jointly with associates of the Pathophysiology Section of the Institute of Experimental Medicine of the Academy of Sciences of the Hungarian People's Republic (headed by Academician E. Stark) by Zs. Ach, K. Abavari, and K. Szalai.

Academician P. N. Veselkin (USSR Academy of Medical Sciences) and Doctor of Medical Sciences Yu. N. Zubzhitskiy took an active part in discussion of the data.

We express our profound gratitude to all our colleagues, who have rendered invaluable assistance in implementing this work.

The immunologic part of the research presented in chapter 3 was conducted by L. M. Khay at the Department of Microbiology of the Institute of Experimental Medicine of the USSR Academy of Sciences under the direction of V. I. Ioffe. The morphological analysis of the brain was carried out by the neurohistologists M. V. Kovalenkova-Medvedeva and I. P. Tsvetkova with the consultative support of A. G. Knorre and G. P. Obukhova, and subsequently under the direction of Yu. M. Zhabotinskiy. We express to them our deep and sincere gratitude.

1 Major Stages in the Investigation of the Influence of the Nervous System on Immune Processes

Great healers and thinkers of antiquity, such as Avicenna and Hippocrates, observing the course of diseases in different patients, understood the significance of the patient's emotional attitude in determining the course and outcome of the disease. In "preimmunologic" times, when the world of microorganisms was not known and ideas about the structure and function of the nervous system were rather vague, it is natural that not even conjecture was possible about a connection between the nervous system and the defense mechanisms against infections.

The science dealing with the connection of the brain and the mechanisms of specific resistance had its beginnings when the effect of transection or extirpation of parts of the brain on the course of the infectious process was demonstrated for the first time by Savchenko (1891) and London (1899).

The idea of elucidating the influence of the nervous system on the development of immune reactions attracted so many investigators that almost simultaneously many variants of experiments were carried out to answer the question in a general form: Does the nervous system influence the course of immune reactions? At this stage the question was not yet about specific mechanisms and details. Rather, by influencing the nervous system in various ways, researchers attempted to modulate its functional state and against this background to study the course of specific defense reactions (antibody formation in most cases). As a rule, substances were used that excite or inhibit the central nervous system (CNS).

5

In general, the investigators reached the conclusion that substances that inhibit cerebral function, including soporific and narcotic drugs, inhibit the immune reactivity of the organism (Germanov 1953; Zdrodovskiy 1969; Uchitel' and Maysyuk 1952) and decrease the phagocytic reaction (Belyavskiy 1958; Sumarokov 1955), the activity of the reticuloendothelial system (Karpov 1952), and the intensity of antibody formation (Kurashvili 1953; Nesterenko 1958; Palant et al. 1955). Electronarcosis produced the same effects (Kurashvili 1953).

It is important to recall the significance of the reports by Strigin (1953) about the importance of the time of administration of soporifics or narcotics in relation to introduction of the antigen. Thus, in experiments with rabbits it was possible to detect the influence of prolonged sleep on the agglutination titer to typhoid vaccine only when sleep was induced at the moment antibodies began to develop. There was no effect when sleep was induced after the production of immune bodies had begun. Narcosis ameliorates the course of anaphylactic shock, as demonstrated by Mats-Rossinskaya (1957). Anodizing the brain (Vasil'yev and Lapitskiy 1944) has the same effect. Different effects and opposite reactions were reported by Firsova (1953) and Budylin (1953).

In several types of experiments on various animal species, the following general principle was demonstrated: stimulating the CNS intensifies immune reactions (Glotova, Vakhmistrova, and Ignatovich 1931). Caffeine, amphetamine, strychnine, and other substances were used as CNS stimulants. Immune responses to the administration of typhoid vaccine, brucellosis allergin, dysentery bacilli, pertussis vaccine, live brucellosis vaccine, and tick-borne encephalitis virus were more intense in stimulated animals than in controls (Mel'nikov 1954; Orlova 1958; Palant et al. 1955; Tul'chinskaya and Aplyak 1955; Fedorov 1965).

Without examining the mechanisms of the effect of the pharmacologic agents or describing the details of the formation of immune responses to particular antigens, we wish here only to emphasize the general conclusions arrived at by most investigators: the level of activity of the CNS and its functional state are of significance for the formation of immune processes in higher organisms; excitation of the CNS stimulates immune processes, whereas inhibition reduces immune activity.

7   Major Stages in the Investigation of the
Influence of the Nervous System on
Immune Processes

In general, by answering positively the question whether the CNS influences immune reactions, these investigators did not pretend to analyze the phenomenon observed, but created a foundation for further research, including study of the effects on immune reactions of ablation of large sections of the brain. The pioneer in this kind of investigation, Savchenko (1891), established that section of the cervical spinal cord makes pigeons susceptible to anthrax, which usually does not affect them. London (1899) showed that a similar effect occurs in pigeons following extirpation of the cerebral hemispheres.

In spite of crude surgical procedures and the "nongradation" of the tests, these investigators demonstrated for the first time the involvement of the brain in the course of the infectious process. Bogendorfer (1927) established in his experiments with dogs that section of the cervical spinal cord had an inhibiting influence on antibody genesis when the operation was performed before or one minute after administration of the antigen; at a later intervention (after 30 minutes to 24 hours) the effect was not observed. Section of the thoracic spinal cord had no influence on the level of antibodies (agglutinins) in the blood.

Removing the cerebral gray matter in rabbits also causes some suppression of antibody production (Vygodchikov 1952). It is difficult to interpret the mechanisms of the effect of such complex and traumatic surgical procedures. For example, Kurashvili (1953) showed that, following section of the cervical spinal cord in warm-blooded animals, the suppression of production of antibodies to the influenza virus results from a drop in body temperature. Investigations conducted in the early 1950s also suggest some correlation between the level of activity or functional state of the CNS and the course of immune reactions. For example, the functional state of the nervous system associated with the development of conditioned reflexes or of orienting reactions increases the intensity of antibody formation (Monayenkov 1956; Pronin 1954).

Under conditions of overstrain of higher nervous activity (experimental neurosis), an inhibition of the development of antitoxic immunity was observed in guinea pigs vaccinated with diphtheria antitoxin (Shtyrova and Stankevich 1954). Similar results were obtained by Pronin (1954).

Volkova-Borzunina (1952) and Pletsityy and Monayenkov (1963) determined the correlation between the type of higher nervous activ-

ity in horses and the character of immune reactions. In horses classified as showing a strong type of higher nervous activity, in contrast to animals showing a weak type, antibody production in the blood (for example, tetanus antitoxin) proceeds rapidly, the titer of antibodies in the blood rises to high levels, and the amount of antigen decreases rapidly (Monayenkov 1970).

The possibility of conditioned reflex reproduction of the process of antibody production deserves special attention. We should emphasize at this point the importance of careful use of terminology and interpretation of data observed in the course of conditioned reflex experiments. One should distinguish between the production of antibodies and their mobilization; if this is not possible, then one should report only changes in level of antibodies in the blood. Meeting these conditions would eliminate a great deal of confusion.

A number of authors (Golovkova 1947; Pel'ts 1955) have reported conditioned reflex reproduction of cell reactions (lymphocytic reactions, leukocytosis, phagocytosis). Belen'kiy (1955) observed in dogs a conditioned reflex change in blood components arising concomitantly with the contraction of the spleen. Experimental study of "immune" conditioned reflexes in various animals, using various conditioned stimuli, not only corroborated the possibility that there is a temporary connection of such kind, but made it possible to characterize it as rapidly developing, stable, and exhibiting slow extinction (Dolin 1951; Dolin and Krylov 1952; Dolin et al. 1963).

In one of the variants of experiments by Dolin and Krylov (1952), binding the paws and immobilizing the animal served as the conditioned signal. It is now well known that this method itself causes a state of stress and changes the hormonal status of the organism so abruptly that many researchers use it as a test for nonspecific reaction of the adrenal cortex. A more appropriate design, which combines light and sound signals with administration of an antigen, made it possible for Mustardy et al. (1954) to observe an increase in the titer of antibodies in the blood by giving the conditioned stimulus alone.

Savchuk (1952, 1955), after triple immunization of rabbits, determined the titer of agglutinins in the blood, then paired an auditory stimulus with the administration of caffeine, which raised the titer of antibodies. He thus demonstrated a conditioned reflex reaction

9   Major Stages in the Investigation of the
Influence of the Nervous System on
Immune Processes

to caffeine. The well-designed experiment of Luk'yanenko et al. (1962) consisted in developing a stereotype to subcutaneous administration of a physiological saline solution to sensitized rabbits. Subsequent administration of an antigen (instead of an isotonic saline solution) did not cause a local anaphylactic reaction. The authors consider that this absence of the classic effect is determined by the influence of the CNS, in particular the presence of an elaborated stereotype.

Years of experimental and theoretical discussion have been devoted to the possibility of a conditioned reflex regulation of immune reactions. The problem has been subjected to extensive experimental investigation and theoretical discussion, in which the following investigators have participated: Ado and Ishimova (1958); Zil'ber (1958); Zdrodovskiy (1969); Dolin and Krylov (1952); and Gordiyenko et al. (1958). Of these investigators, Ado, Zil'ber, and Zdrodovskiy, in contrast to other authors, did not obtain corroboration of the possibility of producing conditioned immune reactions and did not consider it justified to maintain that such a mechanism is present in the regulation of immune processes.

The history of this question and the associated controversy attest to the difficulty of the problem (Vasil'yev 1963). Attempts had been made to investigate conditioned reflex regulation of immune reactions before strict theoretical and methodological bases for its solution appeared. At the same time, this problem attracted the attention of many scientists, which intensified the development of this area of investigation.

One of the main reasons for the difficulty of achieving conditioned reflex reproduction of immune reactions, in particular antibody genesis, is the lack of factual knowledge concerning the mechanisms of regulation of antibody production in the organism. To illustrate this statement we need only name some of the unresolved questions. It is known that the antigen, upon entering the organism, makes contact with the cells of lymphoid tissues, which, after complex transformations, produce antibodies. The process of antibody formation is possible in vitro, though only in the presence of definite biologically active substances. Yet the dynamics of the development of the process in the organism depend not only on genetically predetermined tendencies, but also on the state of the organism. This is

well known and does not require proof; it indicates the existence of some kind of mechanisms providing appropriate situations and a series of specific protective reactions, including antibody genesis. According to one point of view the antigen, once it enters the internal environment, acts on the receptor apparatus responsible for sending signals to the CNS concerning the entrance of a foreign protein (Gordiyenko 1954, 1965; Gordiyenko et al. 1958). These authors suggest that the transmitted signal carries specific information, that is, a message about the character of the antigen entering the organism. This point of view assumes the existence of a receptor apparatus in the periphery that responds specifically to foreign proteins and also the presence of a means of transmitting information on the entrance of the antigen into the organism. Subsequent experiments did not confirm these assumptions (Ado and Ishimova 1958; Oyvin and Sergeyev 1956). There is an opinion that the antigens act on the receptor apparatus but that the afferent message contains information only about the entrance into the organism of a genetically foreign body, not about a particular antigen; that is, the information is not specific in the immunologic sense (Ado 1952; Frolov 1974).

A different position is possible, based on the assumption that the antigen is capable of penetrating the blood-brain barrier and stimulating definite brain areas—for example, hypothalamic structures. Finally, the possibility should not be ruled out that the antigen entering the organism causes the formation in lymphoid tissue cells of substances that are the intermediaries signaling the CNS about the invasion by a foreign protein. These signals can also be transmitted by neural pathways or can directly affect certain brain areas, as is well known now in regard to leukocyte pyrogens (Belyavskiy 1966, Belyavskiy 1958; Veselkin 1963; Repin 1969).

Another difficulty should be mentioned: the process of producing antibodies was, as a rule, studied on animals whose blood already contained antibodies. Subsequently, the administration of antigen was repeated, but combined with a conditioned stimulus, and 15–60 minutes later an increased titer of antibodies was observed. What is the basis for such rapid increase in antibody titer? Is it the production of antibodies, their mobilization from depots, their redistribution, or perhaps hemoconcentration?

The mechanism of peripheral unconditioned reactions is complex and ambiguous. In different investigations different components

11   Major Stages in the Investigation of the
Influence of the Nervous System on
Immune Processes

could predominate. It is difficult to exclude the possibility that in some experiments reflex spleen contraction developed, in others, a decrease in the level of corticosteroids, in still others, a change in the electrolyte components of the blood. Therefore it is not surprising that there are differences in the results of the experiments and their interpretation. There are too many unknowns in the unconditioned reflex link, a knowledge of which is essential in investigating regulatory mechanisms at different hierarchical levels of the CNS. Thus at present conditioned reflex regulation of antibody production has not been proved to exist.

Further investigation of the question can be approached from several directions. One of the basic problems is analyzing the nature of the influence of the CNS on immune processes. Are these regulating influences? From the point of view of control theory, regulating systems of the simplest type can be referred to as having a receptor apparatus, afferent pathways ensuring input about the entrance of antigen into the organism, a central control link (in the CNS), specific efferent pathways for signaling effector organs transmitting instructions to regulatory mechanisms (neural and humoral), effector links (in this case, lymphoid tissue), and secondary feedback or return afferentation that ensures input to the control center about the successful execution of the efferent instruction.

On the basis of this scheme it would be necessary to investigate the following problems: (1) the receptor apparatus for the antigen stimulus; (2) afferent pathways for transmitting to the CNS signals about the antigen invasion; (3) the organization of the CNS control systems for this function; (4) neural and humoral pathways from the CNS to lymphoid tissues; (5) the mechanisms of feedback or return afferentation signaling the successful completion of the efferent "command."

The present state of investigation is such that it is impossible to answer all these questions. The scant literature on the first two points was cited earlier. In this respect the following fact should be emphasized: antigens are a strong, sometimes extraordinary stimulus to the nervous system (Ado 1952), not to mention the situations of sensitization and anaphylaxis leading to the development of not only functional but also organic damage to the CNS (Baydakov 1958; Glazyrina 1958; Rafika 1960; Khozak 1953).

Problems of organization of a system of central regulation, as

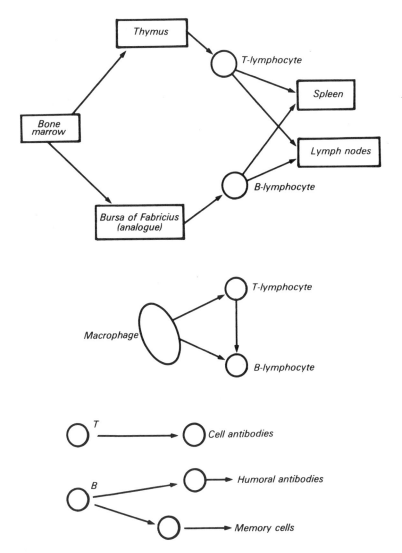

Fig. 1   Schema of the maturation of immunocompetent cells (T and B) and their interactions in the development of an immune response. From Petrov (1976). For explanation, see text.

13   Major Stages in the Investigation of the
        Influence of the Nervous System on
        Immune Processes

now known, will be described along with experimental data. Problems of organization of return afferentation (feedback) have scarcely been investigated in this area.

Scientists have focused primary attention on analyzing the influence of the various sections of the nervous system on the dynamics of immune processes, mainly the process of antibody production and the manifestation of allergic reactions; that is, the presence or absence of the effect of the experimental interventions was judged by the result of the process. Such an approach has its advantages, inasmuch as it lets us evaluate the biological (adaptive) essence of the observed phenomena. However, this approach does not analyze the behavior of different components of the process of immunogenesis, and it leaves open the question about the regulatory mechanisms.

The generally accepted schema of the immune process (fig. 1), while demonstrating the complexity of its organization, at the same time demonstrates the usefulness of investigating the regulation of the different components of the reaction between them as well as their interactions. According to current concepts, an immune process is established through interacting activities of bone marrow, thymus, spleen, and lymph nodes. Some of the stem cells of the bone marrow migrate to the thymus, while others migrate to the bursa of Fabricius in birds or its analogue in mammals (it is assumed they could be Peyer's patches) (Petrov et al. 1975). In these organs the stem cells change and emerge in the form of T- and B-derived lymphocytes, which, after entering lymph nodes and the spleen, lead to the development of cell immunity (T-lymphocytes) and humoral immunity and memory cells (B-lymphocytes) (fig. 1*a*,*c*). Optimal activity is provided by the cooperation of macrophages and T- and B-lymphocytes (fig. 1*b*).

The data on regulation of the components of the process are scant and will be referred to in the appropriate chapters. Unfortunately, their analysis does not permit elucidation of the specific significance of the individual components in the development of the immune process.

2 The Sympathoadrenal System and Immune Reactions

The importance of studying the role of the autonomic nervous system in regulating antibody production was emphasized early by Gamaleya (1928). However, the results of experimental investigations of the influence of the sympathetic nervous system on the dynamics of specific protective reactions have been contradictory.

In essence, investigators have reported all variants of the possible answers to this question, from ruling out altogether the influence of the sympathetic nervous system on the course of immune processes to strongly asserting the existence of such influences inhibiting or activating the process of antibody production. The probable reasons for such wide disagreements may be ascribed to the following circumstances:

1. Different authors used entirely different, often inadequate, methods of influencing the functions of the sympathetic nervous system (e.g., unilateral cervical sympathectomy).

2. There has been virtually no research on the importance of the temporal relations between the administration of antigen and experimental interference with various links of the sympathetic nervous system.

3. In the process of investigation, dissimilar antigens were used: soluble and corpuscular, toxic and nontoxic. This made subsequent analysis difficult.

With the appearance of important works by Kozlov (1968) and Frolov (1974), this whole question has essentially been resolved.

The data reported by different authors should be examined in re-

lation to the type of experimental manipulation performed on the sympathetic nervous system (Ado 1952; Yelizarova 1954). Many have studied the influences of sympathomimetic substances on antibody formation. Thus administering adrenaline lowered the intensity of antibody production (Yefimova and Kalugina 1953; Kurashvili 1955; Ponomarev and Ebert 1956). Other authors reported increases in antibody titer following administration of adrenaline, ephedrine, and Benzedrine (Morgunov 1954; Enenkel and Pedal 1955; Ungar 1955).

Marchuk (1956) and Mel'nikov (1954) reported that amphetamine stimulates antibody genesis. Avetikyan and Melkumyan (1956a, b), in analyzing the effect of amphetamine on agglutinin titer, concluded that amphetamine has an indirect effect on this process. According to them, amphetamine, acting on the central nervous system, led to the accumulation of substances that inhibited the reaction in the test tube. Litvak (1956) did not detect any changes in antibody production against corpuscular antigen in amphetamine-treated rabbits.

Summarizing the data from investigations of the influence of adrenaline on blood levels of antibodies, it should be noted that the results are inconsistent. The selection of adrenaline as a sympathomimetic agent is inappropriate, since adrenaline is rapidly destroyed in the organism, within a few minutes. In essence, one cannot speak about the effects of adrenaline per se, a long and complex process, but only about some nonspecific aftereffects. On the other hand, it is known that adrenaline does not penetrate the blood/brain barrier, that is, it cannot have any direct activating influence on the adrenoreactive elements of the brain. However, its reflex (Vakar 1968) or peripheral influence on tissues sensitive to the effects of the sympathetic nervous system must not be excluded. Moreover, a reflex effect on the central nervous system of an increased level of adrenaline in the blood is made possible by feedback mechanisms. In that case the homeostatic reactions will be directed toward inhibiting the activity of the sympathetic nervous system.

All these variants of the interpretation of the data permit only one conclusion: on the basis of experiments with the administration of adrenaline, one cannot form an opinion either on the role and place of the sympathetic nervous system in providing immune reactions or

on the nature of its influences on these functions. At the same time, these results can be an essential basis for examining the total factual material obtained in the many variants of experimental inhibition or activation of the various links in the sympathetic nervous system.

Even less clear is the formulation of the question in investigations of the effects of transection of the cervical sympathetic nerve (especially unilaterally) on the process of antibody production. It remains unclear what type of model the authors have attempted to construct in making a unilateral transection of the cervical sympathetic nerve stem. Have they tried to eliminate some peripheral sympathetic effects? Or have they perhaps tried to unilaterally eliminate preganglionic connections of the upper middle cervical sympathetic ganglia? Or, on the contrary, have they tried to stimulate these fibers by irritation in the first hours or even days after transection (before fiber degeneration)? Which of these mechanisms predominates in each particular case is unclear, and therefore the results are correspondingly contradictory. Thus the authors, studying the level of blood antibodies to the antigen administered after section of the sympathetic cervical stem, either did not observe an effect (Gordiyenko 1949; Kurashvili 1955) or observed some intensification of antibody production (Kogan 1958). Stimulation of the same nerve in chronic experiments, if conducted during the period of immunization, increased antibody production. If the nerve was stimulated during a decrease in the level of blood antibodies, an increase in titer did not occur (Gordiyenko 1949).

Many investigators have analyzed the role of the sympathoadrenal system on the course of allergic reactions, including anaphylactic shock (Kozlov 1973; Polushkin 1971; Trankvilitagin 1963; Frolov 1974; Chernukh and Tolmacheva 1963; Shatilova et al. 1970; Belasic et al. 1956). The pathogenesis of anaphylactic shock is complex, and in the mechanisms of its development the level of antibodies in the blood and cells plays a role, as well as the antigen/antibody reaction, the amount of biogenic amines secreted during this reaction, and the change in sensitivity of tissues and receptor apparatus. Inasmuch as the mechanisms of anaphylaxis development have no direct relation to the problem under examination, it is not appropriate to discuss in detail the many investigations conducted in this area. This series of questions is thoroughly described in a mono-

graph by Kozlov (1973). It must only be noted that, according to Kozlov's data, stimulating the sympathoadrenal system ameliorates the course of anaphylactic shock, whereas decreasing the influence of the sympathoadrenal system intensifies the anaphylactic reaction. Kozlov suggests that the sympathetic nervous system plays a significant role in the development of anaphylactic shock.

Much attention has been given to the influence of partial injury of the sympathetic nervous system (gangliectomy) on immunogenesis. Thus it has turned out that bilateral extirpation of the superior cervical ganglia has no effect on the development of a pneumonia focus in the lungs of mice (Khay 1956), lowers immunity to dysentery in immune animals (Ado 1957, 1959; Pytskiy 1954), and aggravates experimental endomyocarditis (Aver'yanova 1970). Znachkova (1945) observed an increase in the titer of precipitins and a reduction in quantity of agglutinins in sympathectomized animals. At the same time, it is known that some antigens (for example, influenza A virus) influence the transmission of excitation in the superior cervical sympathetic ganglia in cats and, acting against a background of subthreshold electrical stimulation, cause contraction of the nictitating membrane (Ado 1959; Medvedev 1957).

In investigating how extirpation of the superior cervical sympathetic ganglia influences antibody production, we (Khay and Korneva 1959) proceeded from anatomophysiological data about the functional significance of these ganglia; namely, we examined this link in the sympathetic nervous system as a structure whose main function is to provide the basal regions of the brain and hypophysis with sympathetic innervation.

We know that postganglionic fibers proceed from the superior cervical ganglia toward the cranium and branch out in the region of the cerebral peduncles (Aleshin 1971). Extirpating these ganglia leads to degeneration of some cellular elements in the hypothalamus and to accumulation of neurosecretion ("colloid") in the anterior hypothalamic nuclei, particularly in cells of the supraoptic and paraventricular nuclei, nuclei of the tuber cinereum, and the hypothalamohypophyseal tract. On the basis of these findings, Popjak (1940) emphasized the functional interconnections of the sympathetic nervous system and central structures of the hypothalamus and hypophysis.

Upon stimulating the superior sympathetic ganglia, one observes swelling, vacuolization of the cytoplasm, and a decrease in the perinuclear neurosecretion in the cells of the supraoptic nucleus (Zhukova 1960). These data correlate well with the results from the investigation of the effects of extirpation of the superior cervical sympathetic ganglia on hypophyseal activity. Thus Vyazovskaya (1960) reported that removing the superior cervical ganglia in rabbits increases the secretion of gonadotropic and thyrotropic hormones; stimulating these ganglia has an opposite effect.

Since suppressing the activity of adrenoreactive elements of the hypothalamus does not fully remove the activating effect of sympathectomy, Vyazovskaya concludes that impulses from the superior cervical sympathetic ganglia can influence the hypophysis indirectly (i.e., via the hypothalamus) as well as directly. Stimulating the cervical sympathetic stem increases the release of the hypophyseal hormones, vasopressin and oxytocin, into the cerebrospinal fluid (Gavrilova 1954).

The investigations above demonstrate that the superior cervical sympathetic ganglia exert an influence on basal regions of the brain and hypophysis, and the removal of these ganglia can be considered a probable sympathetic denervation of the hypothalamus and possibly the hypophysis.

The role of the sympathetic nervous system in the function of the endocrine glands has been described in detail by Azhipa (1976). It is important to note numerous observations recorded in the literature about the influence of the sympathetic nervous system on the level of functioning and the electrical activity of various structures of the diencephalon, particularly the hypothalamus (Anokhin 1957; Karamyan 1959; Sollertinskaya 1958; Bonvallet et al. 1954).

Karamyan and co-workers (Van Tan'-an' 1960; Sollertinskaya 1958) investigated changes in the temporal dynamics of the functional state of subcortical structures; they emphasized that the major changes in the activity of the nuclear formations appear not immediately after sympathectomy, but 5–15 days later.

Therefore it appears that in experiments with extirpation of the cervical sympathetic ganglia results will differ depending on the time between the operative intervention and the administration of antigen. Thus some investigators performed the immunization soon

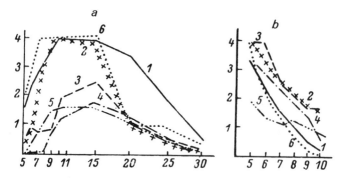

Fig. 2   Dynamics of antibody formation (*a*) and removal of antigens (*b*) in
rabbits at various intervals after extirpation of the surperior cervical sympathetic ganglia: 1, control animals; 2, animals that received
antigen injection 2 days after surgery; 3, 5 days after surgery; 4, 10
days after; 5, 15 days after; 6, 20 days after. Abscissae, time (days)
after antigen was administered; ordinates, intensity of immune reaction (arbitrary units).

after the operation, whereas others began it 2–4 months later, when
compensation for the disturbance may have taken place.

It turned out that bilateral extirpation of the superior cervical
sympathetic ganglia, together with segments of pre- and postganglionic fibers, lowers the intensity of antibody production and suppresses antigen in the blood (fig. 2); the nature of the effect depends
on the time between the operation and the administration of the
antigen. Thus, extirpating sympathetic ganglia 2 days before administering horse serum did not influence antibody production, just as
in the case of sympathectomy 20 days before antigen introduction.
In animals to which antigen was administered 5, 10, and 15 days
after surgery, the intensity of antibody production was lowered and
the disappearance of antigen from the blood was delayed: it could
be detected as long as 10 days after the injection.

These results make it possible to clear up to a certain degree the
cause of the inconsistencies in the literature concerning the influence
of the sympathetic nervous system on immune processes.

As was shown, differences in the results of serological investigations between the experimental and control rabbits were not always
observed, since they depended on the time period between the extir-

pation of the superior cervical sympathetic ganglia and the introduction of the antigen. These differences were marked when this interval was no less than 5 and no longer than 15 days.

It appears that in order to detect distinct changes in the intensity of immunogenesis it is essential not only to surgically exclude the functions of a given neural element, but also to take into account the functional state of other neural centers and structures connected with that part of the sympathetic nervous system. Apparently, 20 days after surgical intervention compensation takes place.

These data do not permit us to determine which stage of immunogenesis extirpation of the superior cervical sympathetic ganglia primarily influences. Inasmuch as production of antibodies is not noticeably lowered when antigen is administered 48 hours after surgery, it appears that by the time the disturbance caused by sympathectomy develops, immunogenesis has already entered its final phase.

Extirpating the cervical sympathetic ganglia most likely affects the initial stage of immunogenesis, which is inhibited and suppressed if the antigen is administered 5–15 days after removal of the sympathetic ganglia. In that case a longer manifestation of the administered antigen in the blood must be regarded as a phenomenon connected with a delay and a less marked so-called immune phase of the process of removal of the antigen from the blood.

The major result of this type of surgical intervention apparently must be considered in terms of its effect on the functional state of neural structures that are under the influence of sympathetic innervation. In this connection, our data agree with the results of investigations cited above (Van-Tan'-an' 1960; Sollertinskaya 1958), to the effect that in rabbits the greatest changes in the electrical activity of the cortex and the hypothalamic region, after extirpation of the superior cervical sympathetic ganglia, arise at the same time as the most pronounced influence on immunogenesis. This permits us to assume that these changes in immunogenesis are associated with the exclusion of the influence of the sympathetic ganglia on the hypophysis, the hypothalamic region, and other basal structures of the brain.

Such an interpretation of these data could be verified experimentally by applying methods of stimulating other links of the sym-

pathoadrenal system, influencing the functional activity of the deep structures of the brain. One experimental design decreased sympathetic influences by removing the adrenal medulla (Korneva and Khay 1961a, b; Khay and Korneva 1961). As is well known, both removing the adrenal medulla and extirpating the superior cervical sympathetic ganglia exert similar effects on the electroencephalogram, conditioned reflexes, cardiovascular system, and other functions (Kibyakov 1950; Sollertinskaya 1958; Yakovleva 1960; Wyman 1929). It is generally considered that the basis for the similarity of these effects lies in their common mechanisms, namely, the effects on the functional state of the hypothalamus and the brain stem reticular formation.

A considerable number of studies of the role of the adrenal glands in protective reactions of the organism did not differentiate between the effects of removing the adrenal medulla and removing the adrenal cortex (Kopytovskaya 1959). Adrenal demedullation was performed electrolytically. At the end of the experiment complete demedullation was verified histologically. In the operated rabbits a delay in antigen disappearance and a decrease in antibody production was observed (fig. 3). This decrease in production was most marked in animals in which antigen was administered 5–7 days after surgery. Thus the results proved similar to those obtained in experiments with extirpation of the superior cervical sympathetic ganglia (Korneva and Khay 1961a, b, 1964).

To characterize the revaccination reaction under the same conditions, the primary immunization (horse serum) was conducted after

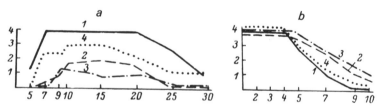

Fig. 3   Dynamics of antibody formation (*a*) and removal of antigens (*b*) in rabbits at various intervals after adrenal demedullation: 1, control animals; 2, animals that received antigen injection 5 days after surgery; 3, 7 days after surgery; 4, 15 days after surgery. Other designations as in figure 2.

demedullation or sympathectomy. Two months later the same antigen was administered in the same dose (0.25 ml/kg) along with another antigen, human serum (0.25 ml/kg). These experiments made it possible to evaluate to what extent the capacity of the experimental rabbits to produce antibodies is restored and to judge the degree of revaccination reaction. The serological response to human serum in the experimental animals was no lower than in the controls, indicating an adequate restoration of the capacity to produce antibodies. Along with this, the revaccination reaction in the operated rabbits was sharply lowered (the titers of antibodies in the control animals exceeded the levels of antibodies in the experimental animals by about twenty times). Thus the primary immunization performed against the background of demedullation or sympathectomy leaves only a faint immunologic trace.

In adrenodemedullated animals, antibody production is decreased and the elimination of antigen from the blood is delayed as a result of this interference; that is, the effects are comparable to those of sympathectomy. Characteristically, the most marked changes were observed if the antigens were introduced not immediately after the surgery, but 6–7 days later. Subsequently the influence of adrenal demedullation on antibody production weakened. Correlation in time and the similarity of the observed changes suggest common mechanisms involved in these effects. Apparently, following adrenal demedullation there is a change in the functional state of the higher vegetative centers, arising as a result of the lessening of activating influences of the sympathoadrenal system.

This assumption corresponds to data in the literature indicating that removing the superior cervical sympathetic ganglia and adrenal demedullation suppress the activity of adrenergic structures of the brain stem reticular formation and hypothalamus (Van-Tan'-an' 1960; Karamyan 1959; Sollertinskaya 1958), although it is difficult to exclude the possibility of peripheral effects of adrenomedullary insufficiency on immunocompetent organs.

Thus a decrease of sympathetic influences produced either by adrenal demedullation or by extirpation of the superior cervical sympathetic ganglia leads to comparable effects. These observations support the idea of a possible central mediation of these influences. Support for such an interpretation of the experimental data is fur-

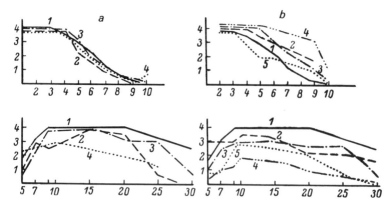

Fig. 4   Dynamics of antibody formation (*lower graphs*) and removal of antigen (*upper graphs*) in rabbits after administration of chlorpromazine (10 mg/kg). *a*: 1, control animals; 2, animals given chlorpromazine for 5 days before antigen administration; 3, 7 days before; 4, 10 days before. *b*: 1, control animals; 2, animals given chlorpromazine for 5 days before antigen administration and for 5 days after; 3, 10 days before and 5 days after; 4, 10 days before and 14 days after; 5, 10 days before and 7 days after. Abscissae, time (days) after antigen administration; ordinates, intensity of immune reaction (arbitrary units).

nished by experiments with chlorpromazine, a substance that has adrenergic blocking effects. Such adrenergic blocking effects on the brain stem reticular formation and hypothalamus were reported by Anokhin (1957), Asyamolova (1958), Biryukov (1958), Val'dman (1958), Mashkovskiy (1956), Shumilina (1956), and Yakovleva (1959). Administering chlorpromazine for 5–10 days (fig. 4) led to a delay in the disappearance of antigen from the blood and to a considerable decrease in the intensity of antibody production (Korneva 1961). It is known that chlorpromazine inhibits adrenergic elements of the hypothalamic region and rostral portions of the reticular formation (Anokhin 1957). However, a possible influence of chlorpromazine on tissue metabolism must also be taken into account (Polishchuk and Vashetko 1958; Berger et al. 1956).

On the basis of these data obtained from experimental exclusion of various links of the sympathoadrenal system (extirpation of the

superior cervical ganglia, adrenal demedullation, chlorpromazine administration), we can conclude that injury to various sections of the sympathoadrenal system or pharmacologic inhibition of adrenoactive structures delays the disappearance of antigen from the organism and suppresses antibody production.

We should emphasize that introducing antigen after suppressing the function of the sympathetic nervous system leaves only a weak immunologic trace. A further attempt to induce a revaccination reaction essentially fails; characteristic dynamics of a secondary immune response does not take place. The reaction is more like that following a primary administration of antigen to the intact animal.

On the whole, the data permit us to assume that the experimental interventions not only exert direct effects on the lymphoid organs but also exert indirect effects by influencing the level of activity of the adrenoreactive brain structures, particularly the hypothalamus and the brain stem reticular formation, which, according to Vogt (1954, 1959), are especially rich in adrenoreactive elements. Therefore it seems justifiable to conclude that inhibiting the functions of adrenoreactive elements of the basal brain structures (which contain central regulatory control elements of the autonomic nervous system) inhibits antibody production and delays the disappearance of antigen.

The results of some physiological experiments support these conclusions. For example, emotional states and reactions to nociceptive stimuli are associated with marked excitation of the sympathetic nervous system and release of adrenaline into the blood (Anokhin and Sudakov 1970; Cannon 1929; Gellhorn 1967). Under such conditions immune reactions are intensified (Gordiyenko 1949). In analyzing the influence of the sympathetic nervous system on antibody genesis, we must also take into account the possible effect of antigen and antigen/antibody complex on the functional state of the central and peripheral divisions of the sympathetic nervous system (Azhipa 1976; Podpolzin 1963; Engelhardt and Lendle 1959). Moreover, as Denisenko and Cherednichenko (1972) mentioned, it is not always possible to distinguish the primary role of each of these influences.

Comparing the literature with results of our own experiments makes it possible to conclude that the sympathetic nervous system very likely participates in regulating the intensity of the immune re-

sponse appropriate for a given antigen. Activation of the sympathetic system stimulates antibody production, whereas inhibition of the level of sympathetic activity is correlated with suppression of antibody genesis and delay in removal of foreign protein.

Thus, the data from the literature do not answer the question of how these influences are exerted, how they reach the effector link of the system (i.e., the immunocompetent cells), whether via neural or humoral pathways. Recent investigations of physiological adjustments of the organism in the process of a reaction to antigen stimulation produced interesting data. Thus Frolov (1974) and Frolov et al. (1972a, b) analyzed changes in the level of blood catecholamines in the process of the reaction to antigen and sensitization. They concluded that the level of catecholamines in the blood at early stages of immunogenesis increases in sensitized animals.

Frolov et al. (1972a) used a successful method of immunosympathectomy that inhibited immunogenesis. Modeling emotional reactions associated with heightened activity of the sympathoadrenal system made it possible to observe a stimulating effect on the formation of immune processes (Makarenko and Frolov 1972; Frolov 1974). All these experimental results allowed the authors to conclude that the predominance of sympathetic regulatory influences stimulates immunogenesis, whereas a decrease in sympathetic regulatory influence suppresses immunogenesis.

Other investigators (Frolov 1972; Frolov et al., 1973) showed the role of the sympathetic nervous system as an effective link in the regulation of immune reactions. Their data agree with the results of recent work on the reaction of lymphocytes to adrenergic substances. It is considered that their effect is mediated via α- and β-adrenoreceptors of lymphoid cells (Golubeva et al. 1975; Hadden et al. 1970; Ladosz 1969). Data demonstrated that the catecholamines not only stimulate phagocytes (Vasil'yev 1963; Gordiyenko 1949), but also increase the mytotic activity of thymocytes (MacManus et al. 1971) and the reaction of blast transformation of lymphocytes in response to phytohemoagglutinin (Hadden et al. 1970). According to data gathered by Ishizuka et al. (1970) and Watts (1971), catecholamines intensify the activity of adenylcyclase in the cells of lymphoid tissue.

In summarizing these data on the influence of the peripheral portions of the sympathetic nervous system on immunogenesis, one can

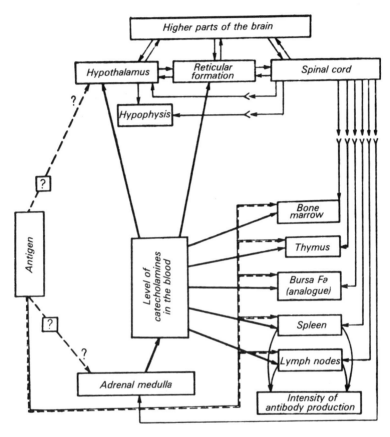

Fig. 5   Participation of the sympathoadrenal system in the regulation of
the intensity of immune reactions. *Thin solid lines,* influences
transmitted by neural elements; *heavy solid lines,* humoral influences; *broken lines,* direct influences of antigens on organs of the
immune system; *question mark,* uninvestigated putative pathways
of antigen influence. Bursa Fa = bursa of Fabricius in birds (analogue of Peyer's patches in mammals).

devise a complex, reasonably clear schema showing how this part of
the vegetative nervous system participates in the regulation of immune processes (fig. 5). The elements of the sympathetic nervous
system innervating the hypophysis and the cerebral peduncle influ-

ence the course of immune reactions, primarily via central brain structures. Together with central brain structures, sympathetic ganglia and nerves innervating the bone marrow, thymus, spleen, and lymphatic glands appear to constitute the efferent pathways that effect immunogenesis. These influences, apparently, are transmitted by catecholamines. Catecholamines activate cell division of thymocytes and lymphoid cells and also stimulate metabolic processes in the cells producing antibodies. If one takes into account that administering antigen increases the level of catecholamines in the blood (i.e., induces a rise in the level of activity of the sympathoadrenal system), then the logical unity of the schema becomes almost complete. Missing are data only on the reaction of the sympathetic nervous system at the time when the titer of blood antibodies decreases—a possible result of the inclusion of feedback mechanisms.

Certain aspects of the influence of the sympathoadrenal system at various stages of immunogenesis have not been investigated. They can be formulated as questions for further experimental investigation:

1. Does the sympathetic nervous system influence the production of stem cells by bone marrow?

2. Are the sympathoadrenal effects important for the process of migration of stem cells from bone marrow to thymus?

3. Does the sympathoadrenal system influence the activity of the thymus?

4. Are sympathetic influences important for the migration of thymus-dependent lymphocytes?

5. Does the level of catecholamines in the blood and tissues play a role in the cooperation of macrophages and T- and B-dependent lymphocytes?

6. How are sympathetic and parasympathetic influences correlated in the regulation of the functions of organs of the immune system?

3   The Influence of the Hypothalamus on Immune Reactions

The study of the role of the hypothalamus in the regulation of specific resistance is historically related to the investigation of other hypothalamic functions. As is well known, the hypothalamus is part of the diencephalon, situated in its basal section. Dorsally it borders on the thalamus; the plane passing through the terminal plate above the optic chiasma serves as its rostral boundary, and its caudal boundary is a plane behind the mammillary bodies.

Macroscopically the hypothalamus is divided into three parts: (1) the anterior part is above the optic chiasma; (2) the midsection, behind the chiasma, is the tuber cinereum, from which the infundibulum begins and stretches to the hypophysis; (3) the posterior part lies caudally from the tuber cinereum, and two protrusions are distinguished in it, the corpora mammillaria. The terms "nucleus" and "area" are most often used to designate the cell concentrations of the hypothalamus. The nuclei are usually isomorphic, the areas heteromorphic (Tsvetkova 1976, 1977). Correspondingly, in all heteromorphic hypothalamic areas the histograms of the distribution of the neuronal contents are polymodal, whereas in the isomorphic hypothalamic nuclei they are monomodal.

In the rabbit, three large groups of neurons extend over the entire length of the hypothalamus in a rostrocaudal direction along the walls of the third ventricle, merging into one another without distinct boundaries and resembling each other in a number of features. These are the medial hypothalamic areas (the medial preoptic area and the anterior and posterior hypothalamic areas), which consist

28

primarily of two types of nerve cells, cytochromic (with an average volume of 450 μ^3) and somatochromic (800–1,000 μ^3) according to Nissl's terminology. These medial areas differ from each other, aside from their topographical position, in their larger or smaller numbers of somatochromic neurons in the main body of cytochromic elements.

The lateral parts of the hypothalamus are occupied by the two lateral hypothalamic areas (the lateral preoptic area and the lateral hypothalamic area), which have no distinct boundary between them in the rostrocaudal direction; along the whole length of the hypothalamus they border on the medial hypothalamic areas. Like the medial areas, they are heteromorphic formations, but their main mass consists of somatochromic neurons (with an average volume of 800–1,300 μ^3), while neurons of another type, small cytochromic (with an average volume of 200–350 μ^3), are found much less frequently.

In the basal part of the hypothalamus are situated the hypothalamic nuclei, each of which consists of one particular type of neuron. The hypothalamic nuclei consisting of small cytochromic elements comprise the suprachiasmatic, the arcuate, the posteriomedial, and the lateral mammillary nuclei, while those consisting of intermediate cytochromic neurons comprise the ventromedial and the medial mammillary nuclei; finally, there is a group of nuclei with somatochromic nerve cells: the paraventricular, supraoptic, supramammillary, and intercalated nuclei. One of the hypothalamic nuclei, the paraventricular, in contrast to the others, lies not at the base of the hypothalamus but in its dorsal part among neurons of the anterior hypothalamic area.

On the basis of these data on the characteristics of the neuronal structure of the various formations of the hypothalamus, Tsvetkova (1977) divides it into three zones:

The medial zone is situated along the wall of the third ventricle and consists of three medial areas: the medial preoptic, the anterior hypothalamic, and the posterior hypothalamic.

The lateral zone occupies the lateral parts of the hypothalamus and consist of two lateral areas, the preoptic and the hypothalamic.

The basal zone is situated at the base of the hypothalamus and includes, in the region of the chiasma, the supraoptic and the suprachiasmatic nuclei; in the region of the tuber cinereum, the paraven-

tricular, ventromedial, posteromedial, and the arcuate nuclei; and in the region of the mammillary bodies, the supramammillary, the medial mammillary, the lateral mammillary, and the intercalated nuclei.

The division of the hypothalamus into medial, lateral, and basal zones presupposes a division in the rostrocaudal direction also, since the areas and nuclei of the hypothalamus, lying in a particular zone, have a definite topographical position with respect to distinct anatomical formations such as the optic chiasma, the tuber cinereum, and the mammillary bodies.

The essential feature of the hypothalamus is the integrative nature of its activity, that is, its regulation of complex functions and processes requiring many components to form an integrated reaction (Tonkikh 1965). This includes homeostatic control of many functions, including temperature, immune reactions, and electrolyte balance, as well as participation in the regulation of emotions, sleep and wakefulness, feeding behavior, and reproduction. The multifunctional nature of this area of the brain should be emphasized: neuronal structures are concentrated here that play a role in the regulation of diverse visceral processes.

It has been shown that the neurons of the hypothalamus respond to afferent stimulation of different modalities (Baklavadzhan 1969; Dafny and Feldman 1970). The ability of hypothalamic neurons to react to changes in the chemical or physical properties of the blood (composition, temperature, osmotic pressure, etc.) is preserved even in surgically isolated parts of the hypothalamus (Aleshin 1971; Polenov 1971; Cross and Kitay 1967). The hypothalamus is a unique neural structure, receiving information about the state of the internal and external environment of the organism through neural and humoral pathways. Whereas individual processes (respiration, heart rate, etc.) are regulated by the lower parts of the brain, the hypothalamus has the property of regulating complex functions of the entire organism in a manner that may be described as homeostatic control.

Since morphologically and functionally the hypothalamus is intimately connected with various brain structures (including limbic structures, cerebral cortex, etc.), in situations of isolation (for example, after surgical intervention), its function is markedly altered (Makara et al. 1969).

As Szentagothai et al. (1965) assume, two possible types of localization of functions coexist in the hypothalamus: the mosaic type (localization of separate processes) and the "general model" type (general functions or types of activity), with the second predominating. This general principle of functional organization provides at the level of the hypothalamus possibilities of inflow and perception of different types of information along neural and humoral channels and with different temporal parameters. Moreover, basic conditions are created that allow compensation for disturbed functions, that is, the ability of the system to maintain homeostatic control.

Elucidation of the role of the hypothalamus in the regulation of vegetative functions, endocrine status of the organism, integration of reactions in the visceral sphere, and maintenance of homeostasis led early to the idea that this area of the brain might participate in the regulation of immune processes protecting the organism from foreign proteins, that is, the preservation of the constancy of its composition. The studies conducted in the thirties in the laboratory of Speranskiy (Speranskiy 1935) were already a direct indication of such a possibility, inasmuch as they attested that the hypothalamus influences trophic processes in the tissues. Furthermore, an increase in sensitivity to saprophyte flora was found upon damage to the hypothalamus, as well as intensification of the reaction to foreign protein (Kanarevskaya 1937).

Between these first investigations, which had formulated the question of the involvement of the hypothalamus in the regulation of immune processes, and the subsequent steps along the way of experimental research, there is a considerable gap, inasmuch as further, more or less continuous development of the problem began in the sixties. By that time a number of indirect data had appeared suggesting the usefulness of experimental research in this direction. Zdrodovskiy, known from his work on neurohumoral regulation of immune processes, concluded that the hypothalamus does participate in these processes (Zdrodovskiy 1969) and developed the theory of the neurohumoral regulation of immune reactions (Zdrodovskiy 1969; Zdrodovskiy and Gurvich 1972).

In clinical studies, data corroborating the influence of emotions and psychological stress on the organism's resistance attracted increasing attention (Kavetsky et al. 1969; Solomon 1969a, b; Solomon et al. 1969); moreover, the observed phenomena were linked

with a change in the functional state of the hypothalamohypophy-seal system, assigning it an essential role in the regulation of specific resistance.

The influence of the hypothalamus on immune reactions was studied by experimental lesions or stimulation of the hypothalamus, beginning with investigations of the process of immunogenesis: the level of antibodies in the blood and the course of anaphylactic shock.

Studies conducted by various authors are not of equal signifi-cance, since some researchers made massive lesions and others made local lesions in various hypothalamic structures. Among the early systematically conducted studies were the investigations by Filipp and co-workers (Filipp and Mess 1969a, b; Filipp and Szentivanyi 1956, 1958; Filipp et al. 1952; Szentivanyi and Filipp 1958), which have shown that massive bilateral lesions of the tuber cinereum in guinea pigs inhibit the development of anaphylactic shock. Control lesions to parts of the cerebral cortex or thalamus or trauma to bone did not have similar effects. The authors emphasized that 55% of the experimental animals died from the surgery and that serious dis-turbances were observed in vegetative and hormonal functions (Fi-lipp and Szentivanyi 1956).

Electrocoagulation of the medial hypothalamus lowers antibody production and alters the antigen/antibody reaction, thus inhibiting anaphylactic shock. At the same time, histamine shock is easily pro-duced in such animals, as are the Arthus and Shwartzman-Sanarelli phenomena. Since injury to the tuber cinereum prevents passive anaphylactic shock as well, these authors (Filipp and Szentivanyi 1958) came to their conclusion about the primary importance of hy-pothalamic influences on antigen/antibody reactions. An attenuat-ing effect on anaphylactic shock was also observed following exten-sive electrolytic lesions of the midbrain reticular formation (Freedman and Fenichel 1958). Lesions of the thalamic structures, operculum, or gray matter of the pons varolii did not have such an effect.

The participation of hypothalamic structures in maintaining non-specific resistance was investigated by Benetato et al. (1945); they es-tablished the influence of the tuber cinereum, mammillary bodies, and lateral hypothalamic area on leukocytosis, which increased

upon stimulation of these cerebral structures. The intensity of the phagocytic reaction is also controlled by the hypothalamic centers; Benetato (1952, 1955) considers this proved, partly on the basis of experiments conducted by the "isolated head" method he developed.

The attempt to analyze the significance of individual groups of nuclei of the hypothalamus in the development of a reaction to foreign protein required the fulfillment of two procedural conditions: a local lesion to the relevant hypothalamic zones and a careful morphological analysis of the location, size, and nature of the focus of the lesion. With limited lesions, one of the most effective sites for modifying immune reactions proved to be the posterior hypothalamic area (Astaf'yeva 1970; Korneva 1964, 1966, 1969; Korneva and Khay 1961a, 1963, 1967; Mikhaylov et al. 1970; Polyak 1968, 1969; Polyak and Bogdanchikova 1967; Polyak and Rumbesht 1968; Polyak et al. 1969; Saakov and Polyak 1967, 1968; Saakov et al. 1976; Solov'yeva 1968).

Experimental manipulation of this area or nucleus (Tsvetkova 1976; Fifkova and Marschal 1962; Sawyer et al. 1954) represents a reasonable model for inhibition or stimulation of immune reactions. In experiments conducted on rabbits, in which various sections of the brain were lesioned, it was possible to observe three types of immune reactions (Korneva and Khay 1961b, 1963): (1) Antigen elimination was markedly slowed, antibody production was depressed, and complement-binding antibodies in the blood could not be detected throughout the experiment (20–30 days) or could be found only in trace amounts (rabbits of group 1); (2) there was a slight inhibition of antibody production and a retention of antigens in the blood (rabbits of group 2); (3) the dynamics of antigen elimination and the production of antibodies were normal or somewhat raised, for example on the 10th day after antigen administration (rabbits of group 3) (fig. 6).

Normally, freeing the organism from a foreign antigen and producing antibodies for a specific dose of antigen proceed rather regularly; the amount of antigen in the blood of rabbits upon intravenous injection of horse serum in a dose of 0.25 mg/kg falls to zero by the 7th–9th day, antibodies appear as early as 5–7 days after administration of the protein, and their number reaches maximum by

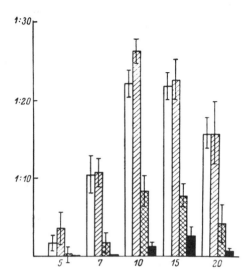

Fig. 6   Dynamics of the process of antibody production in rabbits with hypothalamic lesions: *open bars,* control animals; *solid bars,* animals of group 1; *cross-hatched bars,* group 2; *striped bars,* group 3. Abscissae, time (days) after immunization; ordinates, average antibody titer in blood.

the 15th–20th day, then decreases. Thirty days after administration of the foreign antigen, there are usually few antibodies in the blood, or they have disappeared completely. These changes are characteristic of control (unoperated) animals and of rabbits in group 3. As can be seen from figure 6, the degree of change in the dynamics of immune processes is different in animals of different groups.

Morphological investigation of the brains of these experimental animals has shown that, in rabbits of group 1, the foci of destruction are primarily in the posterior hypothalamic area. Most of the animals of group 2 are characterized by localization of the destruction at the border between the posterior hypothalamic area and surrounding structures, for example, in the ventromedial nuclei of the thalamus and in the subthalamic area; in these cases the zone of destruction extends partway into the posterior hypothalamic area as well. Localization of the destruction was varied in animals of group 3 (fig. 7).

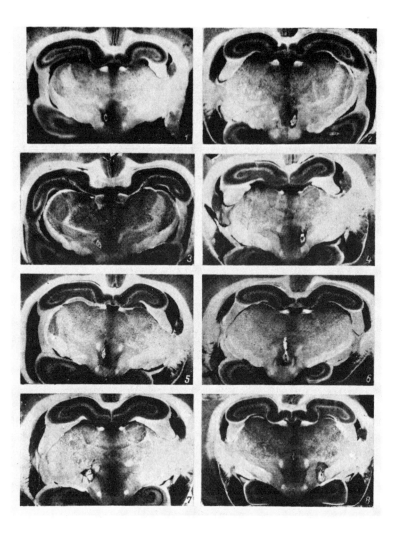

Fig. 7   Lesions of various areas of the hypothalamus in rabbits: 1, in the rostral part of the posterior hypothalamic area; 2, in the ventrocaudal part of the posterior hypothalamic area; 3–4, at the border of the posterior and lateral hypothalamic areas; 5, in the posterior hypothalamic area and the wall of the third ventricle; 6, in the third ventricle and the ventral part of the posterior hypothalamic area; 7, in the lateral hypothalamic area; 8, in the lateral hypothalamic area and the cerebral peduncle.

In the regions of destruction one observes hyperplasia and hypertrophy of glial elements with hypertrophied endothelial cells, and sometimes a periarterial edema with formation of cavities. Fibers of loose connective tissue grow into the damaged tissue areas. On the periphery of a localized lesion, the nerve cells remain without visible changes. Often the foci of destruction involve to a certain extent the wall of the third ventricle; according to serological indicators, the data obtained in these cases are marked by variability.

As was shown by Szentagothai et al. (1965), the walls of the third ventricle are laterally bounded by fibrous structures devoid of cellular elements; this apparently explains to a certain extent the variability of the serological reactions, and often, the absence of any effect. On the other hand, it must be kept in mind that damage to the walls of the third ventricle leads to diverse and often difficult to analyze changes in the humoral makeup of the environment of the hypothalamic neurons.

One should also take into account the possibility of a low immune response in control animals, which in some cases react weakly to the administered antigen (Petrov 1976); this is related to the genetic characteristics of the individual animal (fig. 8).

We examined the correlation of data on localization of the focus of destruction with data on immune indicators. It turned out that most animals with local lesions of the posterior hypothalamic area had poor antibody production, whereas after limited destruction of some other zones of the hypothalamus the immune reactions were close to normal (fig. 8).

An additional form of experimental control was the sequential analysis of the process of antibody synthesis in rabbits before and after surgery. Naturally, in both cases the reaction to the primary administration of several chemically different antigens was investigated.

The morphological structure of the posterior hypothalamic area (Tsvetkova 1976; Nauta 1963) has certain distinctive features. Its main mass consists of small lightly staining cells with a structural organization characteristic of vegetative neurons; they are arranged in groups of three to eight cells. Dispersed over the whole extent of the area are single large cells of the efferent type with large lightly staining nuclei surrounded by a considerable amount of cytoplasm with

The Influence of the Hypothalamus on
Immune Reactions

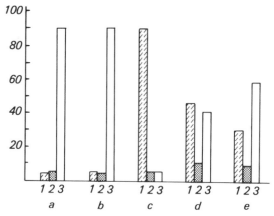

Fig. 8   Histograms of distribution of intensity of antibody production in
control and operated rabbits: *a,* control animals; *b,* experimental
animals with focus of lesion localized outside the posterior hypothalamic area; *c,* with localization in the posterior hypothalamic
area; *d,* at the ventral and lateral borders of the posterior hypothalamic area; *e,* at the border between the posterior hypothalamic
area and the third ventricle. 1–3, groups of animals with different
degrees of immune response (see text). Ordinates, number of animals as a percentage of the total in a given group.

large clumps of darkly staining chromatophilic substance. These
cells are somewhat more often found on the periphery in regions
bordering on fibrous bundles, sometimes forming clusters of two to
three cells. The medial part of the area, around the ventricle, has no
cellular elements.

With the passage of time, the changes in the intensity of immunogenesis, which resulted from injury to the hypothalamus, are restored to normal. Thus, in rabbits that showed marked suppression
of antibody production, the reaction to the administration of another antigen 2 months after surgery was suppressed. After 3.5–4
months the capacity to produce antibodies against the new protein
was restored; the dynamics of antibody formation and elimination
of antigen in such animals was close to normal. If horse serum was
administered for the second time to the same rabbits in addition to
the "new" protein, that is, the same antigen that was administered

immediately after surgery, then in the rabbits of groups 1 and 2 no revaccination reaction was observed; rather, the dynamics of antibody production resembled a primary immune response. Apparently, primary administration of the antigen against the background of a suppressed function of antibody production leaves a weak immune trace, so that the characteristic revaccination reaction to the second administration of protein is essentially not manifested.

The literature includes many data on how hypothalamic lesions influence the intensity of immune reactions. Evidence for the influence on immunogenesis of a more or less extensive destruction of the hypothalamic structures has been obtained in many experiments by administering various antigens (Bogdanchikova 1968; Podpolzin 1963; Saakov et al. 1969; Amkraut and Solomon 1975; Filipp 1971; Jankovic and Isakovic 1973; Konar and Manchanda 1972; Stein et al. 1969). However, there are studies whose results do not agree with those described above. Thrasher et al. (1971), working with rats, observed no effect of injury to the hypothalamus on the intensity of the immune response caused by egg albumin with adjuvant. In these experiments, electrodes were implanted into the comparable zones of the brain in the control animals, which is hardly appropriate, since implanting electrodes per se leads to local destruction and cannot be considered an adequate control. Moreover, in these experiments the precise location of the lesions was not given, but only the zone (the anterior, medial, or posterior hypothalamus). Depending on the location of the focus of destruction within these zones, the effect could differ. Such type of experiment does not make it possible to demonstrate changes in the course of the immune reaction. One also gets the impression that pooled blood from the entire group of rats, rather than separate samples drawn from individual rats, was used in these experiments.

Since the functional organization of the hypothalamus is complex and its structures are heterogeneous, in analyzing the results of studies of this kind it is necessary to make rigorous comparisons of data on immune responses with data on morphological changes and to determine the degree of their correlation. Negative data on the influence of the hypothalamus on immune responses have also been reported in the USSR (Ado and Gol'dshteyn 1974; Gol'dshteyn 1971). These authors maintain that not only the specificity, but also the in-

tensity, of immune reactions is genetically predetermined and not corrected (modified) by the nervous system.

On the basis of our current knowledge concerning the effects of hormones (somatotropin, thyroid hormones, and corticosteroids) on lymphoid cells and on migration and proliferation of stem cells and cells of the thymus, as well as our knowledge concerning the significance of a number of mediating systems (for example, adrenoreactive ones) for the activity of the lymphoid cells, it is difficult to imagine that the structures of the hypothalamus (which regulates endocrine functions and the operation of the sympathoadrenal system) are not involved in the regulation of immune homeostasis.

If we analyze the results obtained from various studies of the effects of lesions of hypothalamic structures on immunogenesis, we obtain a reasonable picture of the study of localization of functions in the hypothalamus in general. It turns out that various investigators using different methods of lesion formation and immunization have succeeded in detecting an influence of the hypothalamic structures on immune reactions. Moreover, if the lesion is massive, damage to almost any zone of the hypothalamus will show this influence (Filipp et al. 1952; Kanda 1959a, b). With clearer delineation of the foci of destruction, as well as in cases of local lesions or irritations, two basic zones can be distinguished that influence specific resistance: the structures of the anterior hypothalamus (Golubeva et al. 1975; Zubzhitskiy and Ogurtsov 1976; Shul'gina et al. 1975; Nauta 1960; Jankovic et al. 1972) and several zones of the medial and posterior hypothalamus, particularly the posterior hypothalamic area.

Some authors (Frolov 1974) have found that stimulating the lateral and the medial regions of the hypothalamus causes opposite effects: suppression or stimulation of immune processes. They attribute this to stimulation of predominantly sympathetic or parasympathetic regions.

According to data by Maros et al. (1960), damage to the reticular structures of the midbrain, situated at the aqueduct of Sylvius, has a unique effect on the relative proportions of plasma proteins, causing a statistically significant lowering of plasma albumin and an increase in gamma globulin. Damage to the ventromedial region of the hypothalamus changes sensitivity to egg albumin (Ado and Gushchin 1965; Ado and Ishimova 1958; Gushchin 1962). Lesions in the

anterior regions of the hypothalamus eliminate the reaction of the adrenal medulla to the administration of foreign blood (Shepotinovskiy 1966).

Studies analyzing changes in the reaction to transplanted skin show that the hypothalamus affects not only humoral but also cellular immunity (Gorbunova 1975; Korneva et al. 1969; Mikhaylov et al. 1970; Solov'yeva 1968, 1969; Tsypin and Mal'tsev 1967; Shepotinovskiy 1966).

In experiments with allogenic skin transplants, an inhibition of rejection for up to 40 days was observed.

Groot and Harris (1950) showed for the first time that it is possible to influence the intensity of immune processes by stimulating the hypothalamic structures. Upon stimulating the tuber cinereum and mammillary bodies, they observed an inhibition of allergic reactions; this was later confirmed by Szentivanyi and Szekely (1956) on a model of anaphylactic shock.

The first investigations of the effect of stimulating the hypothalamus on the titers of already-produced antibodies, conducted on dogs with preliminary immunization with typhoid vaccine or brucellosis antigen, made it possible to observe a stimulating or, at greater current strength, a depressing influence of stimulation of the hypothalamus on the level of antibodies in the blood (Morenkov 1959; Petrovskiy 1961; Khlebutina 1957). The observed changes in the agglutinin levels in the blood were marked (four- to sixteenfold), appeared rapidly (within minutes), and as a rule could be detected over a period of 1–2 hours. Stimulating regions of the cerebral cortex did not cause such an effect. Similar results were obtained by Yegorov (1966), who observed a rise in antibody titers after electrostimulation of the hypothalamus, if it was performed during the final phase of the immunization process, following a decrease in the number of antibodies in the blood (unfortunately it is not indicated which areas were stimulated). Stimulation simultaneous with immunization did not produce the effect.

Contrary to expectations, upon stimulation of the posterior hypothalamic area by electrodes implanted into this area, no stimulation of the process of immunogenesis was observed (Korneva and Khay 1966). In these experiments, electrodes with a small interelectrode

distance were used—that is, a small section of brain tissue was stimulated. The control rabbits had electrodes implanted, but there was no electrical stimulation of the brain. The animals were divided into three groups (1–3) according to the type of disturbance of antibody production and antigen elimination, analogous to the groups of animals with lesions of various brain zones (fig. 6).

It must be emphasized that the results of experiments conducted on rabbits subjected to stimulation and on control animals were similar; that is, the changes in the immune processes occurred whether or not electrostimulation was applied. In the cases where the electrodes ended in the posterior hypothalamic area or passed through it, production of antibodies was depressed whether or not the stimulation was applied. A lowering of the production of antibodies was also observed in rabbits with electrodes passing through the border with the posterior hypothalamic area. At different locations of the electrodes, the dynamics of the immune curves differed little or not at all from normal.

It is of interest to recall the results of experiments conducted by Tsypin and Mal'tsev (1967), who observed a lowering of the titers of normal typhoid O-agglutinins following stimulation of the posterior hypothalamus with chronically implanted electrodes. Some inhibition of immunogenesis upon stimulation of the posterior hypothalamic area was also noticed by Stepanyan (1966) (the unipolar electrode was implanted into the posterior hypothalamus).

Thus, in the nature of the immune reactions, the results under examination coincide with data obtained in experiments involving destruction of various zones of the midbrain. It is possible that the procedure of implanting electrodes into the posterior hypothalamus per se causes such destruction of tissue and thus changes the functional nature of the injured region to such an extent that it suppresses immune processes, and therefore subsequent stimulation with electric current is ineffective.

In a series of investigations we implanted electrodes in such a way that one of them was situated to the front and the other to the back of the posterior hypothalamic area. Inasmuch as the tips of the electrodes were uncovered for 3–4 mm, the current passing between them had to encompass a relatively wide strip of brain tissue and

could pass through the posterior hypothalamic area or bypass it depending on the location of the implanted electrodes (Korneva and Khay 1967).

Such experiments demand a large number of controls, since it is necessary to separate the animal's reaction to the implantation of electrodes from the effect of stimulation with electric current. In this particular case, three types of controls were used: one group of animals was not subjected to electrostimulation, although electrodes were implanted; another control, which made it possible to evaluate the significance of electrical stimulation in the onset of the observed immune changes, was the investigation of the dynamics of antibody production in rabbits before and after stimulation; that is, 5–7 days after implantation of the electrodes the animals were injected with a foreign protein (normal rat serum), and for 10–15 days the dynamics of the immune reactions was traced. Thereafter began daily stimulation with electric current, and 3–5 days later antigens were once more administered to the animals—but antigens of a different type, normal horse serum—and the process of antibody production and antigen elimination was monitored under conditions of continuous electrostimulation. Finally, intact rabbits served as the third control group.

Selecting the parameters of the stimulating current also demands much attention. There are no adequate criteria for correct selection; therefore, in each particular case we chose a threshold or suprathreshold amplitude electric current causing changes in vegetative reactions. The most labile indicators were the EEG of the brain area under investigation, the rate and nature of respiration, and sometimes the heart rate. Stimulation was carried out daily, with a current of 0.5—4.0 V with frequency of 50–100 impulses/sec, applied minutes. Depending on the conditions and purposes of a particular experiment, the period of stimulation varied from 5 to 30 days. The threshold current strength was determined before each stimulation.

The results of the experiments on control rabbits with implanted electrodes but not subjected to stimulation were essentially similar to data obtained after lesions of the hypothalamic structures; that is, in some of the animals immunogenesis was to a greater or lesser degree depressed. In contrast, investigation of immune reactions in rabbits subjected to stimulation revealed four types of reactions:

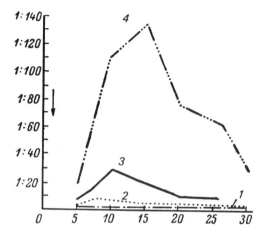

Fig. 9   Dynamics of antibody formation in rabbits subjected to cerebral
                stimulation by means of widely spaced electrodes. *Arrow,* begin-
                ning of cerebral stimulation. 1–4, groups of animals with various
                types of immune reactions. Abscissae, time (days) after beginning
                of stimulation; ordinates, mean antibody titer in blood.

group 1, markedly depressed; group 2, slightly depressed; group 3, not differing from normal; and group 4, definitely increased.

Comparing these data with the results obtained after destruction of various structures of the hypothalamus demonstrates a similarity of the immune reactions in both cases for the first three groups. But stimulation of immunogenesis (rabbits of group 4) is observed only in experiments with electrostimulation of the brain (Korneva and Khay 1967).

As can be seen in figure 9, in animals of group 4 antibodies are detected in the blood earlier than in intact rabbits; their titers are already high on the 5th–7th day. At the height of antibody production, that is, on the 10th–15th day, the antibody titers are higher in rabbits of this group than in control animals, and antibodies in the blood can be detected for a prolonged period: on the 25th–30th day of the experiment they do not as a rule subside, as was observed in control animals.

A comparison of data on serological investigations with morphological verification of electrode placement in animals that were or

Table 1   Dependence of the Nature of the Immune Reaction in Rabbits on the Location of the Stimulating Electrodes

Production of Antibodies in Rabbits	Location of Electrodes			Total Number of Rabbits
	One Electrode in Posterior Hypothalamic Area	One or Both Electrodes at Border with Posterior Hypothalamic Area	Both Electrodes outside Posterior Hypothalamic Area	
With electrical stimulation				
Strongly inhibited	4	1	—	5
Weakly inhibited	—	5	—	5
Unchanged	—	—	—	—
Increased	—	—	16	16
Without electrical stimulation				
Strongly inhibited	1	—	—	1
Weakly inhibited	—	4	—	4
Unchanged	—	—	8	8
Increased	—	—	—	—
Total number of rabbits	5	10	24	39

were not subjected to hypothalamic electrostimulation is given in table 1. The course of the immune process in these animals was determined by two conditions: the location of the electrodes and the factor of stimulation of the brain with an electric current. If the electrodes were placed outside the posterior hypothalamic area and the current passed through this structure (rabbits of group 4), a stimulation of immunogenesis was observed. If, however, the current did not get into the posterior hypothalamic area, there was no rise in antibody production. In the same rabbits the reaction to the administration of a different foreign protein before electrostimulation was normal or somewhat lowered, and only as a result of stimulation was the process of antibody production enhanced, both with respect to rate of appearance in the blood and with respect to the number of complement-binding antibodies. In rabbits not subjected to electrostimulation, no marked increase in immune reactions was ever observed.

As shown by a comparison of the dynamics of antibody formation in response to rat serum administered before stimulation of the hypothalamus and to horse protein injected during electrostimulation of the hypothalamus, stimulation begun 15–17 days after administration of the antigen did not cause an increase in antibody production; the dynamics of antibody formation proceeded normally, and by the 20th–25th day antibody titers in the blood fell to zero in spite of electrostimulation of the hypothalamus. In the same animals, the reaction to horse serum administered 3–4 days after the beginning of electrostimulation of the posterior hypothalamic area increased (fig. 9). Consequently, electrostimulation of the posterior hypothalamus stimulates immunogenesis only if it affects the initial phases of the process of antibody formation. In this type of experiment, electrostimulation encompassed a rather large segment of hypothalamic tisssue, and this must be taken into account in interpreting the data, especially with relation to the precision of electrode location.

A large group of investigations deals with the role of the hypothalamus in the manifestation not of immune reactions per se, but of processes connected with them, for example, the dynamics of tumor development (Garkavi 1962; Ukolova and Bordyushkov 1963; Ukolova et al. 1962). These authors succeeded in demonstrating the existence of a definite influence of the hypothalamus on the growth of transplanted sarcomas and ovarian tumors; the effect could differ, aggravating the tumor or facilitating its resorption, depending on the regimen of the applied stimulation.

Some studies were directed toward determining the influence of hypothalamic stimulation on the course of different kinds of pathologic processes. For example, Zborovskiy and Chistovskiy (1963) observed that electrostimulation of the anterior hypothalamus aggravates the course of streptococcal hyperergic inflammation and intensifies the immune vegetative allergic reactions. At the same time, according to Abinder (1963), stimulation of the anterior parts of the hypothalamus, though not affecting the onset of anaphylactic shock, definitely decreases the number of lethal outcomes. The possibility of producing definite changes in antibody levels in the blood by affecting the hypothalamus is shown in the work of Frolov (1974) and Shatilova et al. (1970); stimulation of the medial hypothalamus

led to a rise in antibody titers, while stimulation of the lateral hypothalamus lowered them.

Thus, changes in the functions of the hypothalamus have an effect on the dynamics of the development of various kinds of immune reactions. The question remains, What are the mechanisms, links, and stages of these influences? According to the schema given by Petrov (1976), several populations of cells participate in the immune process (stem cells, macrophages, T- and B-lymphocytes, antibody-forming cells); therefore it would be of interest to analyze the influence of the hypothalamus on these cellular structures. Such data are lacking with respect to the production and migration of stem cells of bone marrow.

The morphological picture of the lymphoid organs changes after damage to the hypothalamus. From preliminary observations by Martsinkevich (unpublished data), one can conclude that at a later period (after 2 months) the destruction of hypothalamic nuclei affects the system of lymphoid organs as a whole, causing a reduction, first of all, in the B-dependent zones. The intensity of these changes is especially great in the group of animals exposed to the action of antigens before and after the destruction of the hypothalamic nuclei. In this group an increase in the T-dependent zones in the peripheral organs is characteristic, especially in the spleen, accompanied by simultaneous depletion of thymus lymphocytes.

When the antigen is administered after the destruction of the hypothalamic nuclei, the T-zones of the peripheral lymphoid tissue are clearly delineated but considerably less developed. The reduction of the lymphoid tissue in the B-zones is accompanied by a sharp drop in the number of mature lymphoid cells; this is probably connected with changes in the ratio of blast and mature forms in favor of the former. Maturation of cells of the lymphoid line is evidently inhibited, which causes a marked decrease in the number of follicles in peripheral organs. The spleen in such animals looks peculiar at the early stages (3–5 days): the number of follicles in it is increased, but subsequent immunization does not lead to a characteristic stimulation of its activity, at least according to a rough indicator such as a count of the number of follicles in cross sections (Beme, Marat, unpublished data).

According to Khay (1956), the hypothalamus exerts an influence primarily on the first (inductive) phase of immunogenesis and on the process of antigen elimination.

Considering different phases of the immune response, we still need to explain how the changes in hypothalamic functions influence the macrophage phase of the reaction, the proliferation of cells and their maturation, the level of activity of lymphoid and plasmocyte cells, and the cooperation between T- and B-dependent lymphocytes and macrophages.

As a result of highly systematic studies by Shekoyan (1975) and Shekoyan et al. (1975, 1976), it was established that after injury of the posterior hypothalamus the activity of the macrophages is decreased. This decrease is related primarily to their lysosomal rather than their phagocytic functions. This apparently leads to an incomplete transformation of the antigen in the cell. The morphology of the macrophages obtained from such animals and studied by means of a scanning electron microscope changes: the macrophages lose their usual form and become stratified, and vacuoles appear in the cell. In the same experimental animals, antibody production is lowered.

Thakur and Manchanda (1969) and Konar and Manchanda (1970) emphasize that changes in phagocytic activity are especially marked after influences on the medial and posterior areas of the hypothalamus; lesions there lower, and stimulation raises, the activity of the reticuloendothelial system. Highly original experiments conducted by Marat (1971, 1973), Golubeva et al. (1971, 1975), and Shul'gina et al. (1973) made it possible to detect by tissue culture methods changes in macrophage reactions in response to administration of antigens to animals with a damaged hypothalamus and depressed antibody production. Thus all these investigations suggest that the nonspecific macrophagal phase of the development of an immune response may be significant in the implementation of hypothalamic influences on reactions of this kind.

Studies of the proliferation and differentiation of cells of the lymphoid and plasmocyte types in the spleen and lymph nodes after lesions of the posterior hypothalamic area also revealed changes in these processes. Thus, in the spleen of some strains of mice, the

number of sensitized lymphocytes decreased substantially (fifteen-fold compared with control animals). The same is observed in the lymph nodes, although in a less clear form, possibly because in these studies an intraperitoneal immunization was used (Zubzhitskiy and Ogurtsov 1976; Korneva et al. 1969).

Morphological changes in the lymphoid organs were studied in detail in the course of the reaction to antigens following electrocoagulation of structures of the posterior hypothalamus (Kishkovskaya 1972a, b, 1974; Polyak et al. 1975; Rumbesht 1970). In regional lymph nodes and in the spleen, the plasmocyte reaction was depressed; the number of antibody-producing cells was lower on the 5th, 7th, 10th, 15th, and 20th days after immunization; and in the period between the 10th and 20th days the kinetics of the accumulation of antibody-producing cells showed especially marked disruption; possibly this is connected with the depression of the release to differentiation of an additional number of precursor cells, which is characteristic of a primary immune response (Polyak et al. 1975). Morphologically, a predominance of young forms (blasts) has been established among patch-forming cells. The authors attribute this to the retardation of the differentiation of cells of the plasmocyte series. The net effect of the process is that the level of hemolysin in such animals is significantly lowered, in contrast with the hemagglutinins, the dynamics of which are distinctive.

Thus the impression is created that damage to the hypothalamic structures retards the proliferation and differentiation of cells in the spleen and lymph nodes and decreases the number of antibody-producing cells. There are also data suggesting a depression of antibody-forming capacity, in the opinion of Polyak (1969) and Zotova (1968). A recent study by Kishkovskaya (1974), who used histochemical and electron-microscopic methods, corroborated this suggestion. In particular, it was shown that, in rats with damage to the posterior hypothalamic area, the cell reactions in the lymphoid organs and the metabolic processes in the producer cells are depressed. The ultrastructure of cells of the plasmocyte series, in the author's opinion, indicates a lowering of their functional activity.

It is known that comparative data from electron microscopy, especially for such a complex experimental design, must be evaluated with great care. One of the problems is the use of statistical methods

for data verification; however, photodocumentation even by itself is still useful. Thus these results indicate that the modulating influences of the hypothalamus are directed at different and primarily nonspecific components of the immune process, though there also is information about changes in the antibody-forming activity of immunocompetent cells following lesions of the posterior hypothalamic area. Moreover, stimulated and unstimulated cultures of lymphoid cells obtained from the blood of such animals do not show changes; that is, the reaction of the blast transformation of lymphoid cells proceeds in the same manner as that in intact animals (Golubeva and Marat 1972; Marat 1973; Shul'gina et al. 1973).

The question of cooperation between T- and B-dependent cells and macrophages following an experimental manipulation of immunogenesis has undergone little investigation. There are data indicating that the number of macrophagal-lymphoid complexes in the spleen and lymph nodes of animals immunized following damage to the hypothalamus is lowered (Kishkovskaya et al. 1975). Experiments concerning the influence of the hypothalamus on macrophage activity indirectly confirm these data. Thus the impression is created that one of the possible mechanisms of the influence of the hypothalamus on immunogenesis is the nonspecific macrophagal component in the process; another mechanism of the influence of the hypothalamus on immunogenesis could be its effects on the proliferation of cells of the lymphoid series and their differentiation and, finally, on the functional activity of antibody-forming cells.

However, the study of mechanisms of neurohumoral influences on immunogenesis is far from complete. The following questions deserve experimental investigation:

1. What is the influence of the hypothalamus on the production of stem cells by the bone marrow and on their migration?

2. Does the hypothalamus influence the functional activity of the thymus and the migration of thymus-dependent cells?

3. Does the hypothalamohypophyseal system regulate the hormonal function of the thymus?

Although an analysis has begun of other stages of the immune process, to which the neurohumoral transmissions may be directed, it cannot be considered complete. Do influences on the nervous system affect the secondary immune response? As was shown, this is

brought about to a large extent by influence on the development of the primary reaction. If, under conditions of damage to the hypothalamus, the process of antibody production is depressed and few memory cells are formed, then the secondary response will also be weakened (Devoyno 1975; Zotova 1967; Korneva and Khay 1963). Polyak et al. (1975) attribute this to a weakening of the immunomorphological reorganization in the lymph nodes, a decrease in the number of precursor cells, and also a disruption of the process of differentiation of antibody-producing cells.

A number of studies have pointed out the significance of hypothalamic influences for the development of cellular immunity. These include, first of all, experiments with transplantation of various tissues (skin, bone, cornea) under conditions of experimental manipulation of the hypothalamus. In particular, it was established that homotransplantation of a skin flap in guinea pigs after preliminary surgical damage to the posterior area of the hypothalamus proceeded successfully; the flap remained in good condition for up to 40 days—that is, the life of the flap was prolonged (Mikhaylov and Shakharova 1969; Solov'yeva 1968). Similar data were obtained under the same conditions in experiments on rabbits. In such animals the dynamics of the acceptance of a bone homotransplant were unusual; the transplant was accepted faster than in control rabbits, and the course of the process was comparable to the acceptance of an autotransplanted bone (Marakusha et al. 1976).

In experiments on some strains of mice, rejection of a skin transplant was induced by sensitization with streptococcal antigen having a common determinant with the skin (Zubzhitskiy and Ogurtsov 1976). When the same procedure was applied to mice with a damaged hypothalamus, no rejection occurred. The immunofluorescent method showed a decrease in the number of sensitized cells in the spleen and lymph nodes as well as a depression of the level of humoral antibodies in operated animals.

In the opinion of Solomon et al. (1974), damage to the hypothalamus in mice has a predominant influence on the reactions of thymus-dependent forms, that is, on cellular immunity.

Although the advances in postburn corneal transplants following experimental electrolysis of part of the posterior hypothalamic area

(Golubeva et al. 1971, 1975) can formally be regarded as a success of transplantation, the prevention of autosensitization to tissue of the cornea injured by the burn evidently plays the major role in the mechanism of this phenomenon. It is believed that this process determines the development of the second wave of inflammation in burns of the eye and makes corneal transplants more difficult.

There are many studies that use models of central inhibition of immune reactions to analyze the pathogenesis of diseases in whose origin allergic or autoallergic reactions are significant. After damage to the hypothalamus and lowering of the immune reactions, allergic experimental polyneuritis in rabbits was markedly intensified, with a larger number of fatal outcomes than in controls (Konovalov et al. 1971). As it turned out, in this situation the number of complement-fixing antibodies decreased with respect to myelin, but the level of myelinotoxic antibodies (determined in a culture of nervous tissue) did not change (Konovalov et al. 1971; Rodshteyn et al. 1974; Chernigovskaya et al. 1975).

It proved possible to correct the development of autoimmune processes and general collagen diseases by acting on the central modulating mechanisms of the hypothalamus (Ado and Ishimova 1958; Al'pern 1964; Astrauskas 1968; Astrauskas and Leonavichene 1975; Astrauskas et al. 1963; Burykina and Krylov 1975; Vogralik 1966; Gushchin 1962; Zborovskiy and Chistovskiy 1975; Leonavichene and Astrauskas 1975; Polyak and Zotova 1975; Serov et al. 1972; Luparello et al. 1964). Studies demonstrating a change in the mechanisms of nonspecific resistance upon experimental manipulation of the hypothalamus also deserve mention (Polyak et al. 1969; Rumbesht 1970; Rumbesht and Shtokolova 1967; Shekoyan and Khasman 1973).

Thus the spectrum of modulating and regulating influences of the hypothalamus on the specific and nonspecific mechanisms of resistance is rather broad. Through what channels can these influences come about? One of them, sympathetic pathways of transmission, was mentioned earlier. Also possible are parasympathetic mechanisms of signal transmission and shifts to humoral methods of regulation via the hypophysis and endocrine glands. It is known, for example, that the exophthalmic activity of the hypophysis is sub-

stantially lowered in rabbits that show depressed antibody production as a result of damage to the hypothalamus (Korneva and Potin 1970).

At the same time, the role and specific significance of individual hormones of the hypophysis and peripheral endocrine glands in regulating immunogenesis is not clear. Although the influence of hypophysectomy on immunogenesis may fail to be manifested—as was the case, for example, in the experiments of Nagareda (1954)—if one administers threshold doses of antigen such an influence can be demonstrated (Lundin 1960). Clinical data demonstrate well the conclusion that hypophysectomy has less dramatic results than does dysfunction of the hypophysis, when as a result of disruption of the hormonal balance serious diseases develop: acromegaly, hypophyseal cachexia or adiposis, diabetes insipidus, and so on (Grashchenkov 1964; Kakhana 1961).

At present we do not have the necessary data to judge about various pathways of efferent transmission of controlling signals to the immune system, but some specific suggestions for research along these lines can be formulated.

1. Does somatotropin participate in the development of immunogenesis? What is the significance of its interaction with other hormones under these conditions?

2. Are reactions of the hormones of the adrenal cortex manifested in the course of development of the immune response? Does the hypothalamus influence these reactions?

3. Do the hypothalamus and hypophysis regulate the hormonal activity of the thymus?

4. What influence do the hormones of other endocrine glands and their correlation have on the course of the immune process? Does the hypothalamus modulate these hormonal reactions and their interactions?

To elucidate the significance of the deep structures of the brain in the modulation of immune homeostasis, it is also necessary to clarify which biochemical (mediator) mechanisms of the central and peripheral nervous systems predominate in this process. The study of these problems has only begun, but some success has already been achieved.

Most systematically studied has been the role of serotonin-reactive and serotoninergic structures in the operation of the central components of the regulation of immunogenesis (Devoyno 1975; Yeremina 1973). From the pharmacologic point of view, these studies have been well carried out: the functions of the serotoninergic structures were modified by various methods, by pharmacologic action on the synthesis and destruction of serotonin and by damage to the rafe nucleus. The subsequent study of immune reactions has shown that serotonin-reactive and serotoninergic elements of the brain participate in the regulation of immune homeostasis, and stimulating them inhibits the development of immune reactions. Of interest is an observation indicating a transhypophyseal transmission of influences of this kind on immunogenesis: after transection of the stem of the hypophysis, experimental manipulations of serotoninergic elements of the brain do not affect the course of the immune process (Devoyno 1975).

Although the role of the sympathetic nervous system in regulating specific resistance has been studied for a long time and many publications deal with this topic, the specific significance of adrenoreactive and adrenergic mechanisms in the function of the central regulatory mechanisms has essentially not been explained. It is known that cells with this form of mediation participate in the process (Denisenko 1970; Denisenko and Cherednichenko 1972), apparently both in the brain and in the periphery, including at the level of lymphoid cells (Golubeva et al. 1975). As stated above, investigators are inclined to think that excitation of neurons of this type activates immune reactions. However, the possibility that the nature and time of development of reactions vary with the level of organization of the process must be taken into account.

Least systematically studied has been the participation of cholinoactive elements of the brain and parasympathetic nervous system in the regulation of immune homeostasis. One gets the impression that activating this system inhibits immune reactions (Kozlov 1968), although some data contradict this conclusion (Gushchin 1975).

In examining the significance of mechanisms of mediation on the periphery, that is, in the transmission of impulses from the CNS to the effectors, we must deal with reactions of each of the links of the

regulated process (bone marrow, thymus, spleen, lymph nodes, and lymphoid cells) to the separate and combined actions of the various mediators. It is much more difficult to study the biochemical organization of the system in the brain, because most polysynaptic chains in the nervous system are polybiochemical; that is, an experimental manipulation of the metabolism or activity of any mediator can affect the course of any process.

Apparently, the most appropriate approach to studying the biochemical organization of the maintenance of immune homeostasis by the brain would be an investigation of the state of the brain's mediator system as it implements reactions to various antigens, with a parallel analysis of the importance of experimental manipulation of the brain's mediator mechanisms (primarily those of the hypothalamus) for the course of immunogenesis. The biochemical makeup of the hypothalamus has not yet been studied sufficiently, though methods for conducting such research have recently been reported.

The cerebral localization of structures involved in regulating immune reactions of various kinds has recently been substantially clarified. It has become evident that the hypothalamus, the reticular formation, and the limbic system are involved to the greatest extent in the regulation of immune homeostasis. The structures of the hypothalamus that are important in regulating complex homeostatic processes have features characteristic of a field (in contrast to nuclei): the presence of neurons of several types, an abundance of dendrites, extensive connections with various structures of the brain, and, within the hypothalamus, the existence of neurons sensitive to changes in the physical and chemical properties of blood.

In concluding the presentation of data pertaining to the influence of the hypothalamus on immune processes, we should mention once more the uncertainty of the situation: the reality of hypothalamic influences on immunogenesis following experimental manipulation of this region of the brain or its pathology under clinical conditions is evident. However, the question remains: What occurs under natural conditions when the entry of an antigen initiates the development of an immune reaction? Is this part of the brain involved, are its functions changed, and when? What nuclear and area structures participate primarily in this process? Such data would give us more justification to form an opinion on the role of the hypothalamus in regulating immune homeostasis.

4   Neural Hypothalamic Mechanisms in the Development of an Immune Response

It follows from the data cited in previous chapters that injury or stimulation of the hypothalamus influences the intensity of immune reactions. The establishment of these facts is an important step in understanding the nature of the reaction of the whole organism to a foreign protein. Nevertheless, to evaluate the participation of the hypothalamus in regulating reactions of this kind, it is necessary to know that in the development of reactions to the antigen, under natural conditions, the hypothalamic structures are included in the process and change the level or character of their activity. In examining the regulation of immune reactions, it is essential to take into account the participation of afferent, central, and efferent mechanisms of the process.

At present the problem of neurohumoral regulation of immunogenesis cannot be developed further without studying the reorganization of the activities of the nuclei and areas in the central link supporting homeostatic mechanisms in the hypothalamus. Within the hypothalamus are found structures regulating numerous reactions designed for the maintenance of homeostasis and integrating a large input of afferent information. These central mechanisms in the hypothalamus coordinate these reactions and ensure the predominance of particular components.

Electroencephalographic investigations of hypothalamic formations have not revealed specific features characteristic of this area of the brain (Gromova et al. 1964; Brooks 1959; Green and Morin 1953). Attempts to detect by EEG the influence of immune pro-

cesses on the activity of hypothalamic structures have also proved fruitless (Bondarev 1963, 1967; Broun 1969a,b; Gordiyenko 1965; Kiseleva 1960, 1963a,b; Markov 1966; Filimonov 1962). A characteristic feature of these investigations is the study of the dynamics of electrical activity of the hypothalamus in the process of sensitization by inserting one electrode in this brain region. If one takes into account the polymorphism and polyfunctionality of the hypothalamic formations, such attempts to study their reactions to antigen stimulation could not be expected to be fruitful.

Furthermore, the overall electrical activity of the brain is a summated indicator, and therefore investigating it cannot definitively explain how various structures of the hypothalamus interact in providing an immune homeostasis. This was demonstrated in the work of Markov (1966): he reported that, in the process of sensitization, identical EEG changes were recorded in the reticular formation of the brain stem, hippocampus, and hypothalamus.

Investigation of central mechanisms regulating various reactions occurring in the organism both normally and in pathological states (in particular in the development of immune reactions) requires analysis of ongoing long-term processes in the brain. We know that impulse activity of neurons is one of the most useful indicators of the work of brain structures. But to reveal, in the activity of hypothalamic neurons, processes connected with the initiation and course of reactions of immunity, one must first investigate the baseline processes in the neurons of the hypothalamic structures, after which the results of stimulating influences will become apparent. In particular, the neurons of the hypothalamus in a living organism receive and process continuously entering information from all systems of the organism and thus maintain control of homeostasis. In this sense the baseline impulse activity of the hypothalamic neurons is an indicator of their natural functional state.

Indeed, the connection of baseline activity with functional state has already been established in the work of Vvedenskiy (1952) and subsequently supported by many experiments (Golikov 1950; Nasonov 1959). Many studies deal with the nature and interpretation of the baseline activity of the central formations (Beritov 1950; Vasilevskiy 1966, 1968; Grachev and Stepushkina 1968; Lebedev and Lutskiy 1968; Livanov 1965; Smirnov 1956).

Granit (1957) views baseline activity as an important function of the nervous system, reflecting the tonic mechanisms of the central nervous system as well as the periodic changes in activity of individual neuronal units. More recent investigations show the connection of the level of baseline activity with the functional state of the brain. The baseline rhythm decreases or is completely suppressed with deepening anesthesia and is markedly reorganized during other changes in the stimulation of central structures, for example, in epilepsy (Vartanyan 1970; Vasilevskiy 1968; Kostyuk 1960; Shapovalov 1964; Hunt and Kuno 1959).

For the neurons of the cortex, Livanov (1965) showed that an increase in excitability is accompanied by a regular increase in the number of neurons with baseline rhythm. Interpreting the biological significance of baseline activity, many authors (Shapovalov 1964, 1966; Perkel et al. 1964; Poggio and Mountcastle 1963) have shown that the physiological index of the intensity of the responses to external stimulants is determined by the level of baseline activity. As Shapovalov (1966) assumes, this interaction has a definite significance in the coordination and self-regulation of the activity of various neurons. One can accept the assumption of Glezer et al. (1968) that the neuron receiving the impulsation is adjusted to a definite range of intervals between impulses that is determined by the character of the baseline activity. The interpretation of the role of baseline activity and its properties as a mechanism providing regularity in the load of nervous elements deserves attention (Lebedev and Lutskiy 1968).

The informational role of baseline activity remains unclear. Kogan (1964) showed that on the evolutionary scale one can observe regular increases in the arrhythmic impulsation of central neurons. This, according to Menitskiy (1964), reflects the increase in complexity of interneural connections and appears to be one of the major conditions for their optimal functioning. Results of experiments (Mountcastle and Powell 1959a,b) add further evidence for the connection between the baseline activity of neurons and the characteristics of the functional organization of their afferent systems.

Investigation of the impulse activity of hypothalamic neurons began comparatively recently (Cross and Green 1959; Nakayama et al. 1961; Sawa et al. 1959). In the past two decades several hundred bibliographic titles in this field have appeared. However, most of these

reports deal only with the modality of reactions of hypothalamic neurons (Verzilova and Kondrat'yeva 1968; Tolkunov 1968; Anand et al. 1962, 1966; Anand and Pillai 1967; Cabanac et al. 1968); in other cases attempts to quantitatively evaluate the character of impulse activity are limited to the particular properties of neurons within the limits of one particular nucleus: tonic neurons (Baust and Katz 1961), interconnections of impulsation of neurons and sigma rhythm, the effects of drugs and hormones on neuronal activity (Barraclough and Cross 1963; Cross and Silver 1965; Feldman and Dafny 1970; Havlicek and Sklenovsky 1967), and inhibitory neurons in the ventromedial nucleus (Murphy and Renaud 1968).

Reports on the relation of hypothalamic neurons to immune processes are scarce. The investigations by Broun (1969a,b) deserve attention. A change in the activity of a number of hypothalamic formations was established (in particular, the role of the posterior hypothalamic area) in the course of development of experimental tuberculosis. After immunizing animals with a large dose of BCG vaccine, and in rabbits with acute tuberculosis, the author observed an increase in the number of baseline-active neurons in the region of the posterior hypothalamic area and in the anterior hypothalamic region and a decrease in their number in the mammillary region and in medial structures of the central hypothalamus (Broun 1969a). Results obtained from a considerable number of animals turned out to be comparable and statistically significant. A disadvantage of such a method is that it uses only a qualitative evaluation of the state of the neurons, that is, the presence or absence of any impulsation in the cell at a particular time. The author did not investigate changes in the character of neural categories connected with the dynamics of its functional state or the switching of neurons during the development of many hypothalamic functions.

By applying quantitative methods to the study of baseline impulse activity of hypothalamic neurons one can show similar features of the activity of neurons of various sections of the hypothalamus, show the heterogeneity of the neural composition of specific morphological nuclei, and give an objective quantitative characterization of the organization of neuronal activity in these structures. The mathematical techniques of contemporary neurophysiology, widely used to study the activity of neurons of the cortex and other sections of the brain, make it possible to describe the regularities that deter-

mine the periodicity of the categories of neurons (Vasilevskiy 1968; Preobrazhenskiy and Yarovitskiy 1963), the characteristics of distribution of intervals between impulses in the activity of neurons (Narushevichus and Maginskis 1966; Gerstein and Kiang 1960; Hagiwara 1954; Nakayama et al. 1966), and the stability of impulse frequency and parameters of the process of restoring the activity (Zelenskaya and Pyatigorskiy 1968; Tolkunov 1968; Poggio and Viernstein 1964).

A principal significance of quantitative characterization of the impulse activity of a sufficiently large number of neurons of various hypothalamic structures is that it makes it possible, on the basis of these characteristics, to turn to a quantitative description of the functional state of the structures themselves and the interrelations between them. This type of description in turn makes it possible to evaluate changes occurring in them in the course of sustained nervous processes, in particular in the reorganization occurring in the organism after immunization. By comparing statistically reliable characterizations in intact animals and during different periods of immunogenesis one can show the reorganization of the activity of each individual hypothalamic formation, the direction of this process, its intensity, the periods of involvement of its various formations, and its relation to the phases of immunogenesis (Klimenko 1971; Korneva et al. 1971).

The advantages of a directed multivariate investigation of complex dynamic reorganizations of nervous processes of hypothalamic formations in the course of prolonged immune reactions are evident. However, the investigator is confronted by the need to apply very subtle methods and a complex mathematical procedure for analyzing and comparing multiparametric experimental data.

Simultaneous microelectrode recording of the impulse activity of hundreds of neurons over several weeks of development of specific immune defense reactions is ruled out for technical reasons. Consequently, one of the most useful solutions in such situations would be to make a statistical comparison of quantitative descriptions of the parameters of neural activity of hypothalamic structures and their relationship before and during different stages after immunization.

The techniques of microelectrode recording of neuronal activity and of stereotaxic insertion of electrodes in deep subcortical forma-

tions of the brain are described in detail in the literature, and we need not discuss them here. The minimal electrophysiological equipment necessary for extracellular investigation of the impulse activity of neurons is simple—an amplifier with high input resistance (of the order of 10^9–10^{12} ohms), an instrumentation that permits subsequent computer analysis of the parameters of various impulses.

The configuration and amplitude of impulses (recorded extracellularly) of the activity of hypothalamic neurons varies within wide limits. Most often, biphasic positive-negative impulses with an amplitude of 0.8 to 5 mV are registered; less often the amplitude of the spikes reaches 10 mV or higher. Monophasic positive or negative potentials are also observed. Kostyuk (1960) and other authors explain the variety of forms of extracellularly registered spikes as spatial interrelations between the end of the microelectrode and the neuron. Temporal parameters of the baseline impulse activity of the hypothalamic neurons recorded in our experiments are very diverse. According to Vasilevskiy's (1966) classification, a single type of activity can be distinguished that represents individual impulses arising in different sequences. In most neurons considerable variation was observed in the magnitude of intervals between impulses; but there were also neurons with distinctly regular activity (fig. 10). The burst activity represented individual impulses grouped into short high-frequency series of discharges containing 2–7 impulses per burst. The intervals between bursts either were regular or varied within rather wide limits (fig. 11). In group activity in each period of activity of the neurons, the number of peak potentials varied from 4–6 to several dozen individual potentials, separated by longer intervals than during burst activity (fig. 12). However most neurons belonged to a mixed type (fig. 13), and their activity showed regular rhythms, bursts, and groups of various sizes with considerable variability of frequency of the process.

The index of average frequency (7.22 impulses/sec) obtained in our experiments (for more than 2,500 neurons) does not differ from values for hypothalamic neurons reported by Dafny and Feldman (1970) and by Findlay and Hayward (1969). In comparison with data in the literature referring to the frequency of firing of neurons of other regions of the brain of rabbits (Vasilevskiy 1966; Livanov

Neural Hypothalamic Mechanisms
in the Development of an
Immune Response

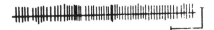

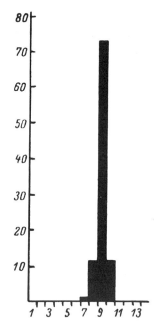

Fig. 10   Histogram of interspike intervals of activity of a hypothalamic neuron (*below*) with single regular type of impulse firing (*above*). Abscissae, numbers of histogram channels, corresponding to a certain
duration of intervals; ordinates, probability of interspike intervals
of corresponding duration, in percent. Calibration: time, 1 sec; amplitude 5 mV.

1965; Melikhova and Shul'gina 1966; Cross and Silver 1963), the activity of hypothalamic neurons is, as a whole, lower. The frequency
of discharges varied from 1 impulse/10 sec up to 10 impulses/sec in
others. Some neurons had an average frequency of discharges in the
baseline activity of more than 20 impulses/sec; however, such activity was rather rare. The magnitude of the average impulse interval,

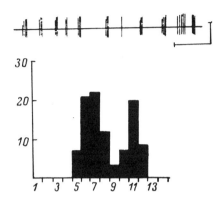

Fig. 11   Histogram of interspike intervals of activity of a hypothalamic neuron (*below*) with burst type of impulse firing (*above*). Designations as in figure 10.

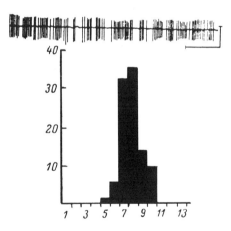

Fig. 12   Histogram of interspike intervals of activity of a hypothalamic neuron (*below*) with cluster (train) type of impulse firing (*above*). Designations as in figure 10.

calculated from all neurons investigated, was 0.139 ± 0.006 sec (which corresponds to a frequency of 7.22 impulses/sec).

Calculations of average values of the frequency of neural impulse activity showed that various structures of the hypothalamus differ from one another according to this index. The zona incerta (Zi) and

Neural Hypothalamic Mechanisms
in the Development of an
Immune Response

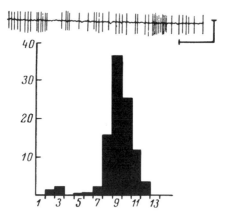

Fig. 13   Histogram of interspike intervals of activity of a hypothalamic neuron (*below*) with mixed type of impulse firing (*above*). Designations
as in figure 10.

ventromedial nucleus (HVM) have the highest frequency; then follow the lateral hypothalamic region (AHL) and the posterior hypothalamic area (NHP). Further in the order of decrease in frequency
are the anterior hypothalamic region (AHA), lateral mammillary
(ML), paraventricular (PV), medial mammillary (MM), supramammillary (SPM), and dorsomedial (HDM) nuclei of the hypothalamus (according to the atlas of Fifkova and Marschal 1962).

   The criterion of the average frequency is one of the mathematical
moments that characterize the distribution of a random value; for
evaluating impulse processes of neurons, investigating the average
number of discharges is clearly insufficient. For instance, many cells
of the visual cortex give a definite response to stimulation of the ret-
ina without changing the average frequency of impulsation; in that
case, the action potentials are simply redistributed in time (Glezer et
al. 1966, 1968; Burns et al. 1962). Much more informative is the investigation of the distribution of the variable value itself, that is, of
the structure of the density of probabilities of distribution of impulse intervals in the analysis of the activity of neurons. The form
and parameters corresponding to the histogram pattern represent
good distinguishing indicators and consequently can be used for
quantitative comparison of the activity of neurons, that is, for their
classification.

However, before constructing histograms of intervals between impulses, one must be assured of the stability of the process. The activity of the hypothalamic neurons has a complex character. Most neurons have a mixed type of activity in which bursts, groups, and single impulses are combined, which makes for a rather large dispersion of the average frequency of impulsation of each neuron. Selecting what segment of the process and what total quantity of the data to analyze is a very important step and can influence the evaluation of the results. Some authors find great irregularity in the impulsation of neurons (Grossman and Viernstein 1961; Rodieck et al. 1962; Viernstein and Grossman 1960); others consider the degree of order in the baseline activity mainly the result of repolarization processes after each impulse (Narushevichus and Maginskis 1966); still others pay attention to the definite periodicity of the activity of neurons in various structures (Andersen 1964; Andersen and Eccles 1962; Levick and Williams 1964). Evidently the periodicity of fluctuations of baseline activity, expressed in various degrees, must be considered a general rule, and cases of simple statistical sequences are probably characteristic of certain relatively short periods of neuronal activity.

The selection of the characteristic impulsation should not depend on the structure of the activity investigated. The evaluation in which time is determined by the number of events and not the number of events by time will be more effective and universal for any configuration of impulse processes. Indeed, if the characteristic is proportionate to the value of 1–2 intervals between impulses, then in the presence of group or burst activity it will change markedly at the transition from intraburst to interburst intervals. The value to be determined must depend as little as possible on maximal and minimal intervals in the sequence examined. According to data by Kulikov (1968), the characteristic based on more than 7–10 sequential intervals includes the evaluation not only of intraburst but also of interburst intervals; that is, it would well describe the impulsation as a whole.

In the investigation of biological processes, methods of analyzing unstable random processes have been applied only recently (Sergeyev et al. 1968). In most cases either the stability was determined visually (Moore et al. 1966) or the constancy of the two first moments—the mean and dispersion—was verified (Alifanov et al.

1968; Kulikov 1968; Cox and Lewis 1969; Rodieck et al. 1962; Werner and Mountcastle 1963). Our investigations have shown that neurons of the hypothalamus under the conditions of our experiment in the course of time intervals of up to one hour do not change the level of average frequency of impulsation or its dispersion and thereby meet the requirements of stability, since the conditions

$$\overline{X}(\Delta t) = \text{const. and } \sigma^2(\Delta t) = \text{const.}$$

are met for all sufficiently large time intervals of the period analyzed (Kulikov 1968; Cox and Lewis 1969). An analogous constancy of statistical characteristics of the activity of central neurons is described by Vasilevskiy (1966) and by Tolkunov (1968). In his monograph Vasilevskiy (1968) writes: "It must be emphasized that any type of activity is stably maintained by each neuron in the course of the whole time of observation (from several minutes to 2–6 hrs), if no sign of injury to the neuron or shift in the microelectrode has taken place."

In view of the great variety of frequency characteristics of hypothalamic neurons, we evaluated the stability of the processes and the construction of histograms according to the number of intervals, not according to a definite time interval. The stability of impulse processes in hypothalamic neurons in our experiments became evident by the time we had analyzed 300 consecutive intervals. Less often it was necessary to examine up to 512 intervals if the process had any stability at all. Usually each histogram was constructed on the basis of 512 intervals. Coding of intervals between impulses and calculation of statistical indexes were done from magnetic recording on a Minsk-32 computer. Histograms of intervals between impulses were constructed for all analyzed impulse processes. The total number of analyzed intervals between impulses was taken as 100%. Thus the weight of channels in the histogram represented the probability of intervals of definite duration, where the first channel contained intervals of duration up to 0.3 msec and each subsequent "k" channel contained intervals from $0.3 \times 2^{k-2}$ to $0.3 \times 2^{k-1}$ msec.

An analysis of the activity of hypothalamic neurons showed that a characteristic form of histograms of the distribution of the duration of interimpulse intervals corresponds to definite types of baseline impulsation of cells. Thus a monomodal form of histogram corresponds to a single type of activity; a bimodal one corresponds to

burst or group types with small spreads of local maxima; and transition forms between bi- and polymodal and equal-probability histograms correspond to the mixed type. The activity of the cell represented by regular impulses following at regular time intervals is represented on the histogram by a maximum in the region of the ninth channel, which corresponds to intervals of 40–80 msec (fig. 10). The dispersion of intervals between impulses is not great, so that the whole mode of the histogram fits into one division of the logarithmic scale of the time axis. Thus, in the case described the histogram of distribution of intervals makes it possible to show rather fully the activity being investigated.

Somewhat more complex is the analysis of bimodal histograms. In figure 11 we can see two clearly defined maxima, corresponding to the high- and low-frequency components of the activity of the cell. It is evident that the activity of the neuron is closest to the burst type of impulsation. An analysis of the form of the histogram of the distribution of interimpulse intervals fully corroborates this conclusion. The first mode is rather wide, occupies four channels, and clearly reflects the variation in the length of intraburst intervals. Using the logarithmic scale of time as a basis for plotting the histograms makes it possible to reflect clearly the considerably smaller variation, relative to the latter, of interburst intervals (the eleventh channel of the histogram).

Where the activity of the neuron groups of impulses (fig. 12) and length of intervals between groups varied to some degree, the histogram mode became more definite, wider, and approached the form of a log normal or exemplary distribution characteristic of truly random processes (Cox and Lewis 1969). The oscillogram shows that the impulses in groups and the groups themselves occur highly irregularly. Figure 13 represents the activity of a neuron of a different configuration. In the histogram of this process the high-and low-frequency components are obviously reflected. The neurogram of the process indicates that this neuron manifests an activity of single group and burst types.

This exhausts the possibilities of visual evaluation of histograms and of the multiparametric indexes of distributions. Obviously, comparing the character of impulse processes of neurons requires a more precise differentiation between similarities and differences of histograms.

Klimenko et al. (1972) developed a method of objective automatic classification of histograms by rank correlation of their attributes— the weight of the channels. According to this method, each histogram is examined as an element possessing a number of attributes. On the basis of the correlations of these indexes, the entire group of elements is divided into classes of histograms that are uniform with respect to a given statistical significance. As a criterion for comparing the histograms they chose Spearman's rank correlation (Plokhinskiy 1970); since the intervals between impulses are distributed according to an unknown law, the histograms are characterized by a relatively small number of parameters (channels), and for analyzing the mutually correlated connection of interval distribution a common and linear correlation of intervals between impulses is of greatest interest.

Analysis by the method of classification described above made it possible to show a number of similar types of distribution of inter-impulse intervals. By nonparametric correlation of channels of histograms whose similarity was no less than 99.9% reliable, thirty-one classes of distributions of intervals between impulses were distinguished. Inasmuch as the histograms within each class are statistically similar, it appeared possible to average them by channels. The means of forms of all classes are shown in figure 14. The values of the average intervals between impulses, dispersion (first and second moments), and average frequency of impulsation for each of the thirty-one classes of distributions are given in table 2. It is of interest that the number of rules determining the structure of the probability densities of distributions of interimpulse intervals of hypothalamic neurons is finite; that is, the regimen of work of the hypothalamic neurons is limited, which can be shown from statistical data accumulation.

Calculations showed that the probability of appearance of a neuron having a distribution of an interimpulse interval of a new, original class decreases exponentially. Its approximation by the function of type $y = \exp(-kX)$ shows that this probability is close to .001 in the investigation of 160–80 neurons of the hypothalamus.

From the literature (Dertouzos 1967) we know that the possibility of using a threshold element as a device of information processing depends on the number of inputs and the value of the threshold. An analogy with the functional organization of neurons comes to mind,

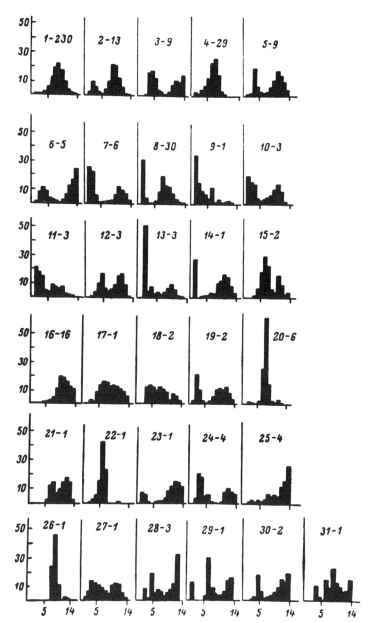

Fig. 14   Types of classes of histograms of impulse intervals. Abscissae, numbers of classes of histograms; ordinates, probability of intervals of corresponding duraiton, in percent. First number above each histogram, class number; second number, number of neurons in the particular class.

Table 2   Statistical Parameters of Classes of Activity of
                 Hypothalamic Neurons

Numbers of Classes of Distributions	Mean Interimpulse Interval (sec)	Error of Mean Interimpulse Interval	Dispersion of Mean Interimpulse Interval	Mean Frequency of Processes (impulses/sec)
1	0.099	0.038	0.142	10.1
2	0.104	0.044	0.191	9.6
3	0.406	0.268	7.051	2.5
4	0.032	0.012	0.015	31.0
5	0.274	0.131	1.665	3.7
6	0.648	0.454	19.920	1.6
7	0.191	0.093	0.793	5.2
8	0.074	0.028	0.076	13.5
9	0.044	0.021	0.038	22.7
10	0.086	0.045	0.191	11.6
11	0.040	0.015	0.020	25.3
12	0.204	0.108	1.146	4.9
13	0.078	0.035	0.122	12.9
14	0.246	0.115	1.279	4.0
15	0.144	0.076	0.516	6.9
16	0.430	0.226	5.000	2.3
17	0.272	0.141	1.846	3.7
18	0.159	0.077	0.572	6.3
19	0.229	0.109	1.162	4.4
20	0.043	0.020	0.043	23.3
21	0.313	0.163	2.646	3.2
22	0.023	0.009	0.008	42.9
23	0.488	0.278	7.602	2.1
24	0.287	0.162	2.669	3.5
25	0.709	0.502	24.923	1.4
26	0.063	0.035	0.101	16.0
27	0.152	0.069	0.472	6.6
28	0.692	0.552	30.300	1.4
29	0.438	0.295	8.286	2.3
30	0.581	0.384	13.283	1.7
31	0.360	0.244	5.926	2.8
Means for all classes	0.139	0.006	0.016	7.2

how it "functions" when the sum of input effects exceeds the value
of the threshold and the number of inputs/synapses is vast. If individual nervous regulating systems are examined, one can be sure
they possess the same properties: a defined threshold of sensitivity

and a large number of inputs. In inherently unstable characteristics, most of the elements would be inefficient, since, if the threshold has a value of several dozens and the inputs are in the hundreds, then errors of transfer coefficients of no more than 1% are permissible. The efficiency of the brain systems (functioning, providing biologically adaptive behavior of the organism) is achieved by periodic participation of all elements in the work of the system. The results of studies by Tolkunov (1968), Vasilevskiy (1968), and other authors, as well as our data, lead to the conclusion that the functional specifics of nervous structures find their reflection not so much in the character of impulsation as in the different correlations of neurons with definite statistical parameters of activity.

The large number of neurons of class 1 is striking. For various structures it constitutes 40–80% of all neurons, and the relation of their number to neurons of other types is constant for each structure. A dispersion analysis of distribution according to hypothalamic neurons of class 1 showed that its structures truly differ in content of these neurons (table 3). This is a basis for assuming that one can judge the dynamics of the functional state of hypothalamic structures by the change in the relation of neurons of class 1 and other changes.

As can be seen in figure 14, the impulse processes of class 1 have a log normal distribution with high dispersion. From the literature we know that truly random processes have such a distribution of variable magnitude (Cox and Lewis 1969). One can only surmise the nature of these neurons and their functional role. For example, they could participate in the activity of various hypothalamic structures as connecting elements; or it is possible that processes of different biological modalities converge on them and that they determine the activity of nonspecific brain systems. A third possibility is that these neurons could be functioning singly ("running on idle") (Kogan 1958, 1969), participating in self-regulation of the level of excitability of structures; as the functional load increases, they could be included in some specific processes.

The distributions of classes 4 and 16–18 approach that of class 1 but follow somewhat different rules. In the distributions of classes 9, 13, 20, 22, and 26 the excess is clearly expressed. Clearly bimodal are the distributions of classes 2, 3, 5–8, 10, 12–14, 19, 23, 24, and

Neural Hypothalamic Mechanisms
          in the Development of an
          Immune Response

Table 3   Statistical Reliability of Difference between Structures according
               to Their Content of Class 1 Neurons

	A	B	AB	X	Z
η	0.001	0.250	0.234	0.485	0.515
σ^2	0.152	5.387	5.047	4.951	0.131
F	1.159	41.146	38.542	37.808	—

Note: A, factor of content of class 1 neurons; B, factor of neuron belonging to a particular structure; η, weight of influence of factor; X, factors not taken into account; Z, randomness factor; σ^2, dispersion; F, Fischer's criterion (index of statistical reliability).

30. A calculation of indexes of asymmetry and excess is obviously not appropriate, since most distributions are not monomodal. A detailed comparison of histograms of interimpulse intervals has shown the existence of a nonparametric correlation of distributions of intervals in the activity of neurons of various hypothalamic structures.

The data cited above make it possible to classify all neurons recorded in hypothalamic structures according to their membership in a specific class. A map was drawn of neural spectra of hypothalamic structures based on the regimen of work of the neurons of each of the morphological formations investigated (fig. 15). The diagrams reflect types of activity of the neurons represented in specific structures and the specific weight of each type. One can see that the preponderance of neurons investigated in each structure have distributions of interimpulse intervals of class 1. With less weight but also found in almost all structures of the hypothalamus are neurons that have distributions of interimpulse intervals belonging to classes 4, 8, and 16. Representation of other classes of neurons in hypothalamic structures has a more complex character, and comparing structures according to parameter 31 (corresponding to the specific class) is visually impossible. Obviously, to solve this problem it is necessary to determine the correlation of neural compositions of the investigated structures and the similarities and differences of functional organization of their activity.

The most adequate method of comparing the data is, in our opinion, factor analysis (Nebylitsyn 1960; Savchuk 1952). It is based on the calculation of the correlation matrix of all elements investigated. Each element is examined according to connections with all the other elements simultaneously and with each separately. Then the regu-

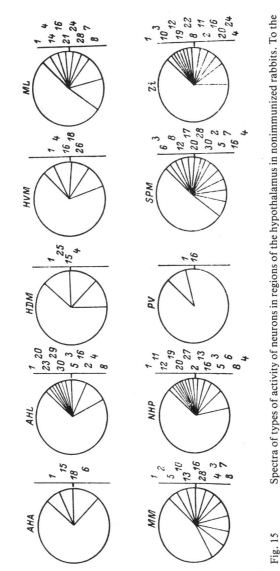

Fig. 15   Spectra of types of activity of neurons in regions of the hypothalamus in nonimmunized rabbits. To the right of the diagrams are the class numbers of the histograms of impulse intervals corresponding to sectors of the diagrams. AHA, anterior hypothalamic area; AHL, lateral hypothalamic area; HDM, dorsomedial nucleus; HVM, ventromedial nucleus; ML, lateral mammillary nucleus; MM, medial mammillary nucleus; NHP, posterior hypothalamic area; PV, paraventricular nucleus; SPM, supramammillary nucleus; Zi, zona incerta.

larities (factors) that stipulate the interconnections in the correlation matrix are mathematically calculated. Thus the matrix of the factor coefficients of the correlation is the result of factor analysis and reflects the character of causes (regularities of observed measurements of differences and similarities of elements), their hierarchy (weight of factors), and the degree of connection of the elements according to their characteristics.

This type of analysis, being an integral statistical method of evaluating the functional organization of complex dynamic processes, is at present widely used in physiological investigations (Bekhtereva et al. 1971; Bundzen et al. 1971; Gogolitsin 1975; Nebylitsyn 1963; Chtetsov 1969; Holm and Schaefer 1969).

There are several types of factor analysis connected with different methods of calculating the factor matrix. We chose the method of main components (Bedretdinov et al. 1969) because (1) the connection between attributes by which the factors are calculated is not known beforehand, which is necessary for group methods (Teplov 1965; Thurstone 1953); (2) there were no hypotheses relative to the distribution of variables, as is proposed in the centroid method and the method of greatest likelihood (Ganenko 1969); (3) this method is easiest to algorithmize for a computer (Klimenko and Kaplunovskiy 1972). The method of main components involves finding the eigenvectors and eigenvalues of the correlation matrix.

Through factor analysis it became clear from the character of the organization of neuron activity that some hypothalamic structures are highly correlated with each other and that there are a number of rules (factors) common to these structures. Three factors carry sufficient weight to merit investigation; the others are unimportant and can be ignored. The first of the factors, F_1 with a maximum weight (96%), fully connected the structure of all studied nuclei (fig. 16). It appears that this was reflected in a wide representation in all nuclei of class 1 neurons as well as those of classes 4, 8, and 16. The second factor, F_2 (weight 1.8%), distinguished common features of the organization of activity of the lateral hypothalamic area (AHL) and medial (MM) and lateral (ML) mammillary nuclei, as well as a negative (with respect to them) correlation in the activity of neurons of the dorsomedial (HDM) and ventromedial (HVM) nuclei, because in these structures the classes of neurons are also less variable in regard to other correlations. The third factor, F_3 (weight 0.8%), re-

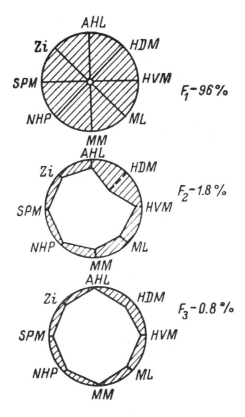

Fig. 16   Interrelations in the organization of neuronal activity of the hypothalamic structures in nonimmunized rabbits. F_1-F_3, connections
according to factors 1–3, respectively; *solid lines*, positive correlation with corresponding factor of connection; *broken line*, negative
correlation. The size of the striped field reflects the degree of manifestation of the given connection. Other designations as in figure
15.

flected a particular interconnection in the activity of neurons of the
dorsomedial and medial mammillary nuclei and a negatively corre-
lating activity of neurons of the ventromedial nuclei.

These data, though they do not make it possible to connect the
known regularities with specific biological reactions in the hypothalamus, do show what is common as well as what is different in the

organization of the activity of this integrated formation of the brain and the interconnection of its morphological structures. These data also represent quantitative characteristics of impulse processes of hypothalamic neurons and create a basis for further comparison of the regimens of work of the neurons in the various structures of the hypothalamus in the course of development of prolonged reactions of specific immune responses (Klimenko and Kaplunovskiy 1972).

As an antigen in the model of immune reactions in rabbits, we used heated "native" (freshly obtained) horse serum in a single intravenous injection of 0.25 ml/kg. The use of "native" serum prevents side effects of toxic substances used to preserve the serum; heating was necessary to destroy complement. In selecting the horse serum as an antigen we were guided first of all by the comparability of the results with data obtained from investigations of the influence of damage and irritation in the hypothalamus on the level of antibodies in the blood of the animals. Antibodies in the blood were determined by the reaction of bonding the complement (prolonged bonding in the cold) in a modification of the method of Ioffe and Rozental' (1943).

On the basis of the well-known character of the immune response of rabbits to the injection of horse serum, we selected the 1st, 3d, 6th, 10th, 15th, 20th, and 30th days after injection of antigen to investigate processes of rearrangement in the central link—the structures of the hypothalamus. In these experiments we studied the activity of neurons of the same ten structures of the hypothalamus as in the nonimmunized animals. In processing the results of observations obtained from each of these periods, we carried out stages of analysis as described above. Histograms of interimpulse intervals and their classification showed fifty-two classes of distributions of intervals between impulses, with their similarity within each class no less than 99.9% reliable (Student's quantile, 4.3). It turned out that thirty-one classes of distributions coincided fully with classes determined during the classification of histograms of interimpulse intervals in neurons of nonimmunized animals; and twenty-one classes of histograms differed from them. The means of all fifty-two classes are depicted in figure 17. The values of the mean interval between impulses, dispersion, and mean frequency of impulsation for each of the fifty-two classes of distributions are shown in table 4.

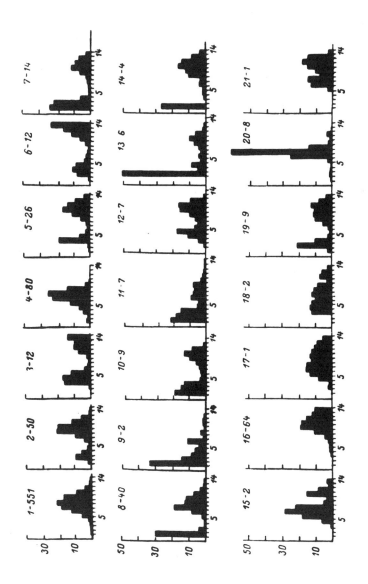

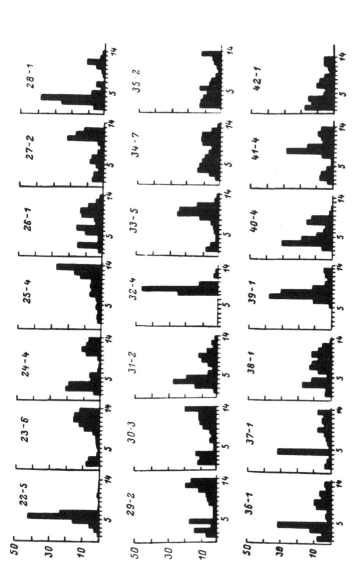

Fig. 17   Types (centers) of histograms of intervals between impulses. Designations as in figure 14.

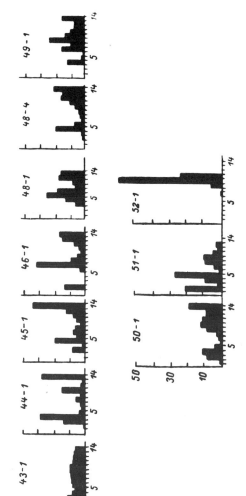

Fig. 17 (*continued*)

Table 4		Statistical Parameters of Classes of Activity of Hypothalamic Neurons		
Numbers of Classes of Distributions	Mean Interimpulse Interval (sec)	Error of Mean Interimpulse Interval	Dispersion of Mean Interimpulse Interval	Mean Frequency of Processes (impulses/sec)
1	0.099	0.038	0.142	10.1
2	0.104	0.044	6.191	9.6
3	0.406	0.268	7.051	2.5
4	0.032	0.012	0.015	31.0
5	0.274	0.131	1.665	3.7
6	0.648	0.454	19.920	1.6
7	0.191	0.093	0.793	5.2
8	0.074	0.028	0.076	13.5
9	0.044	0.021	0.038	22.7
10	0.086	0.045	0.191	11.6
11	0.400	0.015	0.020	25.3
12	0.204	0.108	1.146	4.9
13	0.078	0.035	0.122	12.9
14	0.246	0.115	1.279	4.0
15	0.144	0.076	0.516	6.9
16	0.430	0.226	5.000	2.3
17	0.272	0.141	1.846	3.7
18	0.159	0.077	0.572	6.3
19	0.229	0.109	1.162	4.4
20	0.043	0.020	0.043	23.3
21	0.313	0.163	2.647	3.2
22	0.023	0.09	0.008	42.9
23	0.488	0.278	7.602	2.1
24	0.287	0.162	2.669	3.5
25	0.709	0.502	24.923	1.4
26	0.166	0.072	0.522	6.0
27	0.240	0.140	1.870	4.2
28	0.079	0.050	0.250	12.7
29	0.487	0.306	9.232	2.1
30	0.496	0.341	11.370	2.0
31	0.072	0.032	0.104	14.0
32	0.063	0.035	0.101	16.0
33	0.172	0.082	0.671	5.8
34	0.152	0.069	0.472	6.6
35	0.289	0.221	4.733	3.5
36	0.140	0.069	0.486	7.1
37	0.274	0.180	2.473	3.6
38	0.121	0.061	0.363	8.2

Table 4 *(continued)*

Numbers of Classes of Distributions	Mean Interimpulse Interval (sec)	Error of Mean Interimpulse Interval	Dispersion of Mean Interimpulse Interval	Mean Frequency of Processes (impulses/sec)
39	0.145	0.073	0.545	6.8
40	0.028	0.016	0.025	35.7
41	0.272	0.147	2.147	3.7
42	0.092	0.056	0.309	10.9
43	0.226	0.124	1.532	4.4
44	0.514	0.448	20.680	1.9
45	0.692	0.552	30.300	1.4
46	0.438	0.295	8.286	2.3
47	0.058	0.036	0.124	17.2
48	0.581	0.384	13.283	1.7
49	0.360	0.244	5.926	2.8
50	0.512	0.358	12.706	2.0
51	0.035	0.016	0.027	28.7
52	0.133	0.092	0.801	7.5

It should be noted that the thirty-one classes of distributions common for all series of investigations include 97.1% of all investigated neurons, while newly determined classes have one or two neurons, and their weight amounts to only 2.9%. The appearance of new classes of distributions of interimpulse intervals can be explained, first of all, by the increase in the volume of selection. It is also possible that as a result of immunization the rearrangement of the central regulating systems determines the appearance of new classes.

According to the results of classification, we constructed spectra of neural activity for the hypothalamic formations for each of the studied periods of immunogenesis (fig. 18). The diagrams reflect the types (or classes) of activity of the neurons represented in specific structures and the specific weight of each type of impulsation.

Of special interest are the dynamics of neurons of class 1 in the structures having log normal distribution with high dispersion, or an exponential distribution of interimpulse intervals characteristic of truly random processes (Cox and Lewis 1969). In nonimmunized animals they constituted 46–80% of all neurons of various structures (fig. 15), and the relation of their number to neurons of other types was constant.

Neural Hypothalamic Mechanisms
in the Development of an
Immune Response

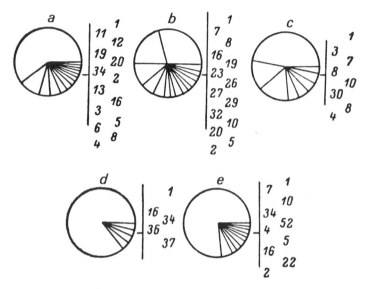

Fig. 18   Dynamics of changes in the activity spectrum of the posterior hypothalamic nucleus in rabbits in early stages of immunogenesis: *a,*
nonimmunized animals; *b-e,* on the 1st, 3d, 6th, and 10th days
after immunization. To the right of the diagrams are the class numbers of the histograms of interimpulse intervals corresponding to
sectors of the diagrams.

This correlation of the activity of neurons in the course of immunologic rearrangement changes within the organism (fig. 18), to different degrees for individual structures. This becomes especially obvious at the earlier periods of immunogenesis. Figure 19 shows the
change in the number of neurons in the structure of the hypothalamus; they have types of distribution of interimpulse intervals different from those of class 1. Note that maxima of changes in almost all
structures are in the initial period (1–3 days) of the development of
immune reactions. As we mentioned above, this period corresponds
to the inductive phase of immunogenesis and is characterized by the
presence of an antigen and by the absence of antibodies in the blood.
As yet there is no specific humoral protection; nevertheless it is important to note marked changes in the neuronal activity in hypothalamic structures during this period. Maximal changes of the value of

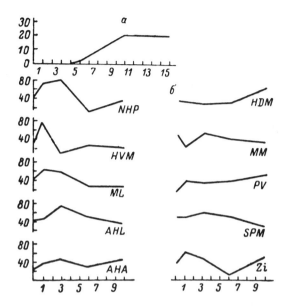

Fig. 19   Dynamics of antibody titers in the blood of rabbits (*upper graph*), and number of neurons in ten hypothalamic structures (*lower graph*) with distributions of interimpulse intervals differing from log normal, during early stages of immunogenesis. Abscissae, time (days) after immunization; ordinates in upper graph, antibody titers; ordinates in lower graph, relative number of neurons, in percent. Other designations as in figure 15.

indicators develop in the activity of neurons of the posterior hypothalamic area and the (morphologically) adjacent region of the ventromedial and lateral mammillary nuclei.

They encompass the whole period of the inductive phase, and later on the curves have a form characteristic of the well-known physiological phenomenon of "return" or, technically speaking, reregulation. By the 10th day the initial correlations of the neurons of the first and the other types of activity are restored to the initial level.

As we pointed out above, local injury to the posterior hypothalamic area, in contrast to the injury to the rest of the hypothalamic formations, suppresses the function of antibody formation. Korneva and Khay (1963) showed that, for the suppression of this func-

tion after immunization, the destruction of the posterior hypothalamic area is effective only during the inductive phase. On the other hand, experiments with electrostimulation of the posterior hypothalamic area (Korneva and Khay 1967) permit us to conclude that the stimulation of immunogenesis is observed only when the stimulation affects the initial phases of the process of antibody formation. Comparing these data with results of the present investigation, described above, leads to the following conclusion.

That maximal changes observed in the activity of neurons of precisely the posterior hypothalamic area correlate with the development of the inductive phase of immunogenesis fully corresponds to data from the literature and confirms the role of the neurons of the posterior hypothalamus in the central regulation of antibody formation. The period of maximal changes in the neural activity of the posterior hypothalamic area is characterized by a marked decrease in the relative number of neurons having a log normal distribution with high dispersion of interimpulse intervals. At the end of the inductive phase, with the appearance of circulating antibodies, the number of neurons of this type increases markedly; thereafter (by the 10th day) it returns to the initial level. It is possible that, in agreement with the view of Kogan (1958, 1969), these neurons work in an "idling regimen," participating in self-regulation of the level of excitability of the structures, and that after massive immunization, as the functional load of the structures increases, they are incorporated in special processes. Figure 20 depicts the dynamics of the number of neurons in the investigated structures of the hypothalamus having types of distribution of interimpulse intervals differing from log normal. It is useful to compare the processes occurring in various structures on one graph, because the general character of the reorganization shows up in greatest relief and encompasses all studied sections of the hypothalamus. These processes end on the 10th day. According to data on serological investigations (Korneva and Khay 1961b, 1963), this period of reorganization corresponds to the conclusion of processes of binding and removal of the antigen from the organism.

Thus, at the first comparison of the dynamics of impulse activity of neurons of various hypothalamic structures in the course of immunologic reorganization occurring in rabbits with the indexes of

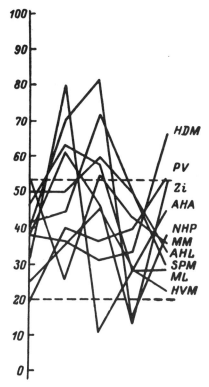

Fig. 20   Dynamics of change in the correlation of types of activity of neurons in hypothalamic structures of rabbits during early stages after
immunization. *Horizontal broken lines,* initial levels of neuronal
activity. Abscissae, time (days) after immunization; ordinates, percentage of neuronal activity with distribution of interimpulse intervals differing from log normal. Other designations as in figure 15.

immunogenesis, interconnections of these processes are already revealed; moreover, it appears that the reactions of the hypothalamic
structures have an individual, unique character. To show the processes of reorganization of neural activity occurring in the hypothalamic structures on all fifty-two parameter classes is a more complex
problem. It requires a specific mathematical treatment.

  To begin with, we must provide a quantitative description of the
interconnection in the organization of the activity of hypothalamic

Neural Hypothalamic Mechanisms
in the Development of an
Immune Response

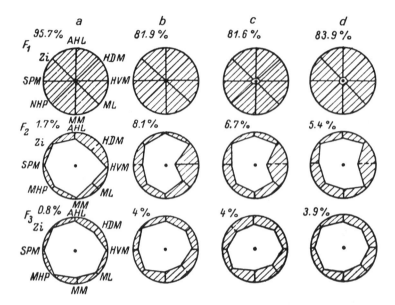

Fig. 21   Interrelations in the organization of neuronal activity of hypothalamic structures in rabbits during early stages after immunization: *a*, control animals; *b*, 1 day after immunization; *c–d*, 3 and 10 days after immunization. The numbers are weights of factors, in percent. Other designations as in figures 15 and 16.

structures for each of the investigated periods of immunogenesis. To solve this problem we calculated matrixes of mutual correlation of hypothalamic structures according to their neuron components during all observed periods of immunogenesis. Investigating the matrixes by factor analysis permitted us to represent graphically the characteristics of interconnection in the activity of the structures at each period of development of immune reactions (fig. 21). It turned out that, as in nonimmunized animals, the general character of neural activity of the various structures is on the whole similar: the first factors with the greatest weight incorporate structures during all stages of immunogenesis. In particular, according to the first factor one can note only a decrease in the specific weight of a given regularity in the organization of the activity of the structure immediately after immunization and a gradual restoration of the initial correla-

tion by the 30th day. The dynamics of the specific weight of the second and third factors show the appearance of new regularities, and their structure reflects a sequential involvement of various formations in the reorganization taking place in neural activity. The observed changes as a whole are also completed by the end of the period of observation.

To analyze the character of reorganization of neural activity in each of the investigated hypothalamic formations, we calculated coefficients of correlation of states (composition) of the structures in nonimmunized animals as well as in animals during different stages of immunogenesis. The obtained correlations of matrixes were investigated by factor analysis (fig. 22).

The dynamics of factor coefficients of correlation illustrate clearly the periods, intensity, and structure of reorganization of neural activity in hypothalamic formations; in particular one can note that each structure differs in periods and direction of reorganization of neural activity. The results of analysis of the interconnection in the organization of the activity of the hypothalamic structures and the description of the dynamics of the composition (neural spectra) of specific structures in the same period make it possible to characterize the changes occurring in the investigated complex of hypothalamic formations in each period and in the course of the whole investigated period of immunogenesis. In the established changes of activity of each hypothalamic structure, we can distinguish two components of reorganization. The differences between them show up when we compare the correlations between the activity of any structure and the activity of other structures during the same periods with the correlation of the activity of the same structure in different periods of immunogenesis.

Thus, in the process of the reaction, the connections of any structure with the rest of the structures changed essentially (the first component of the reorganization of activity). Hence in a number of cases the high degree of connection of organization of its activity remained in the initial state and in the following periods of investigation. In other cases we see the reverse: the second component changes (i.e., the activity in the structure in the subsequent period differs from that in the preceding), and the connection of activity of a given structure with the others (the first component of changes in

Neural Hypothalamic Mechanisms
in the Development of an
Immune Response

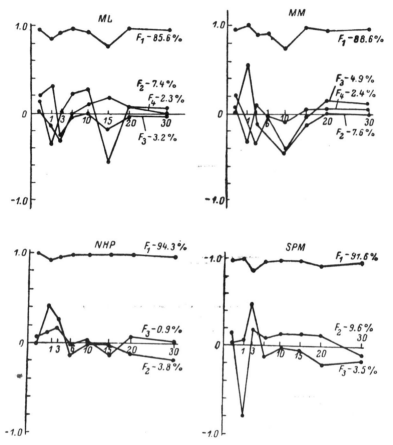

Fig. 22   Principles of reorganization of spectra of neuronal activity of hypothalamic structures. F_1–F_4, factors 1–4 of reorganization; the
weights of the factors are indicated in percent. Abscissae, time
(days) after immunization; ordinates, values of correlation coefficients. Other designations as in figure 15.

activity) remains unchanged. Thus at this stage of analysis it is possible to have a quantitative description of two components of the observed reorganization of the neural activity of hypothalamic structures. The first of these characterizes the interconnection of the
neural activity of any structure of the hypothalamus with that of the

rest of the structures during each of the investigated periods after immunization. The second component reflects the dynamics of the organization of the activity of each of the specific structures in the course of the whole period of observation.

To explain the regularities of the reorganization of the functional organization in the individual structures and in the investigated complex of structures as a whole, we have constructed a graph of the dynamics of indexes of both components of changes of the activity of hypothalamic structures (fig. 23).

On the basis of the description of the dynamics of activity of the hypothalamic structures and their interconnections, we can proceed to a quantitative comparison of the parameters of reorganization of the activity of these structures. Factor analysis is approrpriate as a method of classification (Adam and Enke 1970; Buss and Buss 1970; Overall and Williams 1961). Comparing (fig. 24) the data for the whole period of observations made it possible to arrange the structures in the correlation area according to the similarity of the dynamics of their organization (on the abscissae) and the dynamics of interconnection of their activity (on the ordinates).

This demonstrates that the reorganization in only two of the investigated structures (the posterior hypothalamic area and the supramammillary nucleus) proceeds similarly in the course of the whole period of immunogenesis. This is of great interest, since an analogous construction for comparing the dynamics of reorganization of the activity of hypothalamic formations during early periods, up to 10 days after immunization (fig. 25), clearly illustrates the similarities of the processes (positions in the correlation field) of change in the functional organization of activity in the posterior hypothalamic area and the mammillary, lateral, ventromedial, and supramammillary nuclei. The character of the changes in other structures of the hypothalamus distinguished them from one another and from the formations enumerated above, which determined their individual position in the correlation field. The main graphs in figure 23 are a model including the totality of data obtained on the changes in activity of individual structures, and they make possible a description of the dynamics of the reorganization of the activity of the hypothalamus as a single system. Indeed, the state of the whole system of the complex of the structures under study is characterized first by

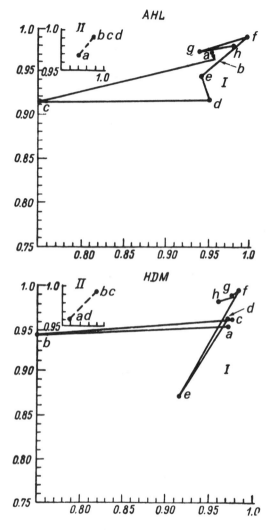

Fig. 23   Dynamics of reorganization of the activity of the hypothalamic
structures and interconnections of their activity in rabbits after administration of horse serum (I) and own serum (II). Points *a–h*
show the position of structures in the correlation field at various
times of immunogenesis: *a,* before immunization; *b–h,* on the 1st,
3d, 6th, 10th, 15th, 20th, and 30th days after immunization. Abscissae, factor correlation coefficients of the activity of the structures; ordinates, factor correlation coefficients of the interconnection of the activity of the structures. Other designations as in figure
15.

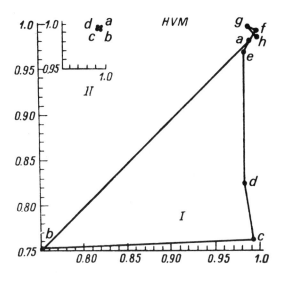

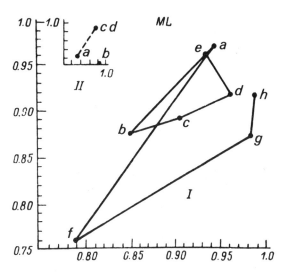

Fig. 23 (*continued*)

90

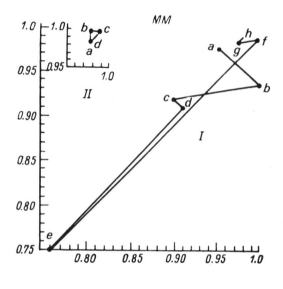

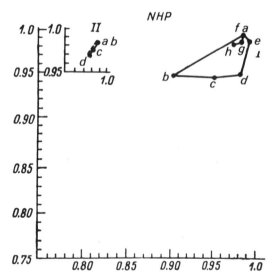

Fig. 23 (*continued*)

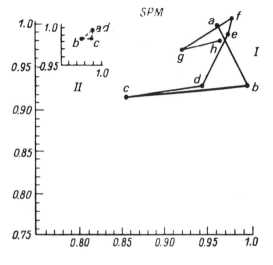

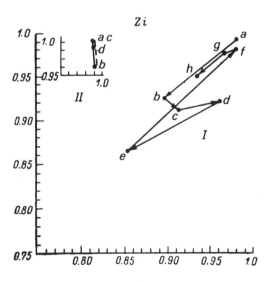

Fig. 23 (*continued*)

Neural Hypothalamic Mechanisms
in the Development of an
Immune Response

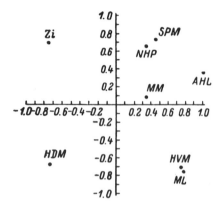

Fig. 24   Connection of processes of rearrangement of neuronal activity of
hypothalamic structures in rabbits in the course of immunogenesis.
The position of the structures in the correlation field is due to the
nature of the change in their activity and the dynamics of the interconnections with the activity of other hypothalamic structures.
Designations as in figures 15 and 23.

the large number of states of its elements (i.e., individual structures)
and second by the large number of indexes of the interconnection of
these elements. The data in figure 23 make it possible to compare the
state (organization) of the hypothalamus at various periods of immunogenesis. Projections of the points corresponding to the periods
of the dynamics of activity of the structures, on the abscissae, give a
series of coefficients characterizing the state (organization) of the
hypothalamus at various periods.

The second aspect of the characteristic of the whole system concerning the dynamics of interconnection of individual structures is
shown upon analogous comparison of the projection on the ordinates of points corresponding to specific days of immunogenesis for
different structures. The correlation of a series of these points reflects changes in the interconnection between the structure of the hypothalamus during the whole investigated period of immunogenesis. Calculating mutual correlations of the series of points and
investigating them by factor analysis makes it possible to reflect

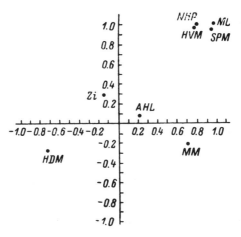

Fig. 25   Connection of processes of rearrangement of neuronal activity of
                hypothalamic structures at early stages (1st–10th days) of immuno-
                genesis. Designations as in figures 15 and 24.

quantitatively the connection of states of the hypothalamus during
various periods of immunogenesis. The results of factor analysis of
the dynamics of correlation connections of the structures are represented in figure 26.

In the resulting reorganization we see that in the period of the inductive phase (1st–3d day) there is a synchronous reaction of structures, since the character of activity of each of them changes, but the
interconnection in the organization of their activity remains. By the
6th day the reaction becomes distinct for each of the investigated
structures, and the index of interconnection changes markedly. By
the 10th day after immunization we see a return of the indexes to the
initial value, and this period corresponds, according to immunologic indexes, to the completion of the removal of the antigen from the
organism. However, by the 15th day we can once more see a return
to the reorganization observed in days 1–3. It is of interest to remember here the dynamics of immune indicators. The removal of antigen
is completed by the 10th day, and the titers of antibodies that increased up to the 15th day begin to decrease. These data permit us to
hypothesize a reflection of mechanisms of inhibition of antibody
synthesis in accordance with feedback principles. In the period of

Neural Hypothalamic Mechanisms
in the Development of an
Immune Response

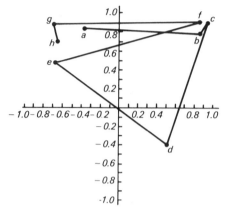

Fig. 26   Dynamics of rearrangement of the functional organization of the
activity of the entire studied complex of hypothalamic structures in
the process of immunogenesis. Designations as in figure 23.

20–30 days after immunization the activity approaches the initial
state.

Before summing up this investigation it seems appropriate to describe the control experiments we undertook to define more precisely, on the same model, the influence on the activity of hypothalamic
structures that do not exhibit antigenic properties. For this we used
the serum of experimental animals, drawn from a vein 2 weeks before the beginning of our neurophysiologic investigation. All other
conditions of the experiments, including the heating of the serum
and the dosages, were identical to those described above. For comparison, the graphs of rearrangement of the activity of the hypothalamic structures in control experiments and in the experiments involving antigen are given in pairs (fig. 23). The scale of the graphs is
the same, but for convenience the graph of reorganization of the activity after administration of nonantigenic serum is placed to the
left. The differences of the reorganization of the activity between the
two are evident. This variant of control experiments, verifying the
connection of the observed changes with the reaction to the antigen
effect, has shown that it is the immunization itself that causes the
marked reorganization of the activity of hypothalamic structures.

Thus this research revealed the changes in the activity of neurons of all investigated structures of the hypothalamus after immunization and let us separate the elements of different importance in the system of central regulation of reactions to antigens.

By studying the dynamics of the process we can separate periods of maximum reorganization, and these maxima are also observed in the inductive phase on the 15th day after immunization. Data on immunologic investigations (Petrov and Zaretskaya 1965; Adler et al. 1966; Bernett 1971) also attest to the intense development of cell reactions in the lymphoid tissue precisely in the inductive phase. Local injury to the posterior hypothalamus inhibited antibody formation only when the surgery was conducted before the introduction of antigen; that is, the effect is also related to the inductive phase of the process.

Among all the links of the system we can see a clearly expressed complex of structures: factor analysis has shown the correlation of processes of reorganization of neuronal activity over the first 10 days after immunization in the region of ventromedial, supramammillary, and lateral nuclei and in the posterior hypothalamic area. According to data in the literature, damage in the area of these first three nuclei does not lead to a marked inhibition of immune reactions. It is therefore logical to assume that the processes in these structures, coinciding with the dynamics of reorganization of neural activity of the posterior hypothalamic area, are essential components of the system that regulates immune reactions of the organism.

It appears that the reactions of hypothalamic formations have systems characteristics and that neurons of all investigated structures of the hyothalamic area are involved in ongoing reorganizations. This is natural, since the intimate cell mechanisms of immunity demand from the organism a reorganization of many nervous and humoral influences, creating conditions for normoergic reactions to a foreign protein and providing a nonspecific reactivity of the organism as well as the intensity of immune responses. This makes it possible to consider appropriate the application of multistage mathematical analyses of neurophysiological indicators reflecting reorganizations of processes in the hypothalamus as well as functional reorganizations of multilink systems in response to the introduction of a foreign protein into the organism.

On the basis of our experimental data and mathematical analysis,

one may conclude that the functional characteristics of hypothalamic structures can be adequately described statistically in experiments on untreated rabbits as well as rabbits responding to an antigen. The possibility of such a description is experimentally and mathematically corroborated by the following basic facts: (1) all observed types of impulsation of hypothalamic neurons could be divided into a finite number of classes: the probability that a new, original class will appear decreases exponentially. Thus the impulse activity of hypothalamic neurons, in spite of the diversity of its variants, can in principle be described by definite regularities, the framework of which predicts any possible manifestations of activity of the cells of the hypothalamic structures under normal and experimental conditions. (2) From this generalization it follows that it is possible to characterize the impulse activity of individual structural and functional parts of the hypothalamus by statistically determined types (classes) of impulsation that are characteristic for neurons of corresponding structures.

As calculation shows, an increase in the number of investigated neurons, although capable of adding something new to the characteristics obtained (for example, that a new, rarely met type of activity is detected), will in principle not change the functional characteristics.

In conclusion, as a result of our investigations it is possible to describe statistically the character of impulsation in neurons of various hypothalamic formations under various conditions. Basic connections and interactions were revealed from the analysis of impulsation of hypothalamic neurons, indicating a definite organization of the processes under study and their reorganization in the course of reactions to antigens. It must be emphasized that the changes detected in the activity of the central nervous system begin before antibodies appear in the blood. Our data establish that hypothalamic structures help regulate the functions controlling immune reactions. However, the question of the mechanisms involved in regulating these functions remains to be studied. At present, we are only in a position to develop hypotheses on the nature of these mechanisms. The most probable suggestion is that integrated nervous and endocrine efferent links participate in this regulation, inasmuch as these central modulating influences appear to be multidirectional and long lasting.

5   Hormones and the Immune Response

As was shown in the preceding chapters, in the intact organism the immune response cannot occur only within the framework of the autonomically functioning and self-regulating system of immunocompetent cells; it also depends on a whole series of neurohumoral factors that determine the condition of the internal environment of the organism. Among the many humoral agents that can influence the course of immune reactions, hormones and neuromediators need to be examined first of all.

The problem of interaction between the immune and endocrine systems has attracted investigators since the beginning of the century. Even then, interesting observations were made indicating that various hormones influence the development of immune reactions. It was established that excluding the functions of endocrine organs as well as administering hormones can change the immune response. Properly, these data served as premises for the concept of possible neurohumoral regulation of the immune reaction together with the existence of mechanisms of specific self-regulation (Zdrodovskiy 1962). Indeed the endocrine system, inseparably connected with the nervous system in function, sensitively reacting to any deviations in the state of the internal environment of the organism by changing the production of hormones capable of influencing all types of metabolism, probably cannot but have a bearing on processes developing in the organism in response to the introduction of antigens. However, the specific ways endocrine factors participate in the development of immune reactions and their role in the course of these reactions have not yet been sufficiently investigated.

98

At present considerable (though in many cases contradictory) experimental material has accumulated on the influence of exogenous hormones on various indicators of immune processes; certain mechanisms of their effect on immunocompetent cells have been established. However, the effects of administering exogenous hormones, often used in large doses, in connection with low toxicity do not reproduce exactly the mechanisms of endogenous hormonal shifts observed under physiological conditions. Therefore special research is needed to elucidate the role of endogenous endocrine factors in regulating immune responses in the intact organism. Thus far two procedures have been used to solve this problem: studying the influence of stress, and excluding the functions of endocrine glands by surgical intervention in the immune process. Apparently, because disturbances of endocrine balance caused by these procedures are so complex, in both cases contradictory results were obtained. Changes in the level of hormones accompanying the development of an immune response have not been extensively studied. At the same time, neuroendocrine shifts in the dynamics of development of the immune process, the study of their correlation with indicators of intensity of normal or pathologically changed immune reactions, and the influence of changes in endocrine hormonal balance on the course of these reactions are especially important in clarifying the interaction of specific and nonspecific factors in the formation of immune responses and in determining the role hormones play in regulating immune homeostasis. In connection with this, we investigated the influence of glucocorticoids.

At present it is difficult to form a complete concept of the role of the hormonal system in regulating immunogenesis. Therefore in this chapter we will attempt to analyze the possibilities and character of participation of only certain individual endocrine factors, based on data currently available on how exogenous and endogenous hormones influence immune reactions.

Hormones of the Hypophysio-adrenocortical System and Immune Processes

In studies of the interrelations of endocrine and immune processes in the organism, the hypophysio-adrenocortical system has

attracted attention for several decades, in view of its important role in the organism's adaptation to the environment (Selye 1952, 1972). At the same time, data accumulated on the influence of adrenocorticotropic hormone (ACTH) and hormones of the adrenal cortex on immune reactions are in many cases contradictory, presumably owing to differences in the experimental models of immune reactions used, to different hormonal preparations, and to different methods of applying them. In particular, the role of endogenous ACTH and of corticosteroids in the development of immune responses has not been sufficiently well investigated.

The Influence of Exogenous Hormones of the Hypophysio-adrenocortical System on Immune Reactions

The effect of exogenous ACTH and corticosteroids on immune reactions has been studied in more detail. It is well established that administering ACTH and glucocorticoids to an organism in large enough doses inhibits the humoral immune response. This effect has been demonstrated in frogs, mice, rats, rabbits, dogs, and humans (D'yachenko 1966; Yekhneva 1975; Kopytovskaya 1970; Meshalova 1958, 1959, 1961; Sergeyev et al. 1971; Uchitel' and Khasman 1968; Chebotarev 1965; Berglund and Fagraens 1961; Darrach 1959; Ducor and Dietrich 1968; Hayashida and Li 1957; Newson and Darrach 1954; Ruben and Vaughan 1974; Szabo et al. 1975).

The inhibiting effects of corticosteroids depend on their chemical structures. Only hormones of the glucocorticoid group, characterized by the presence of oxygen in the eleventh position of the C ring in the steroid molecule (hydrocortisone, corticosterone, and their synthetic analogues) have an immunodepressive effect; mineralocorticoids do not inhibit the synthesis of antibodies; they may even increase it (Gurvich 1963; Zdrodovskiy 1962, 1969; Chebotarev 1965; Ambrose 1970; Shapiro 1957). Most authors agree that the glucocorticoids (hydrocortisone and corticosterone) exert approximately the same degree of inhibition on immune reactions.

The glucocorticoids are capable of suppressing not only the primary but also the secondary immune response (Kopytovskaya 1970;

Shemerovskaya 1974; Eastman et al. 1974; Fischel et al. 1952; Moeschlin et al. 1952). The intensity of the inhibiting effect of glucocorticoids on humoral immune reactions depends on the dosages administered. To depress the humoral immune response, rather large doses of hormones are necessary, up to tens or hundreds of times the physiological levels (D'yachenko 1966; Zdrodovskiy 1969; Sergeyev et al. 1971; Ambrose 1970; Berglund 1956a,b; Darrach 1959). Administering ACTH or glucocorticoids in insufficiently large doses does not inhibit the synthesis of antibodies (Zdrodovskiy 1969; Biornbol et al. 1951).

A number of investigators had difficulty suppressing antibody production in humans, even with large doses of hormones (Hammond and Novak 1950; Larson and Tomlinson 1951; Mirick 1951). However, it is possible that this is connected with insufficient activity of the preparations used. Relatively small doses of ACTH and glucocorticoids apparently can stimulate the humoral immune responses (Ivanov 1963, 1964; Meshalova 1961; White and Goldstein 1970). In carefully controlled experiments Ambrose (1964, 1966, 1970; Ambrose and Coons 1963) established that glucocorticoids, in concentrations approximating physiological range, not only do not inhibit the humoral immune responses in tissue cultures but, on the contrary, are absolutely necessary for a normal course of immune reactions. In the model Ambrose used for studying secondary immune responses of fragments of rabbit lymph nodes to various antigens in a serum-free medium, these concentrations constituted 0.1–1.0 μmole of hydrocortisone, which corresponds approximately to the range of concentrations under physiological conditions. Higher as well as lower concentrations lowered the level of hemagglutinins. In the absence of glucocorticoids the secondary immune response did not appear. Similar data were obtained by other investigators (Brighenti and Gioelli 1966; Halliday and Garvey 1964a,b).

The effectiveness of ACTH and glucocorticoids on the production of humoral antibodies depends to a considerable degree on the antigen dosage and its immunogenic properties. The more closely the dosage of antigen approaches the optimal concentration (i.e., the concentration causing maximal immune response), the larger the dosage of hormone must be to suppress this process. Immune reac-

tions caused by weak antigens are more susceptible to the inhibitory effects of the hormones (Darrach 1959; Ducor and Dietrich 1968).

The intensity of the influence of glucocorticoids on the humoral immune response depends in large measure on when they are applied relative to the moment of immunization. Most authors agree that these hormones cause the most marked inhibition of antibody formation if they are used before immunization or within a few days after it (Meshalova 1961; Sergeyev et al. 1971; Shemerovskaya 1974; Berglund 1956a,b). According to some reports, the glucocorticoids are most effective when they are administered several hours before immunization (Ducor and Dietrich 1968). This gives reason to assume that the inhibiting influence of hormones on the humoral immune response is connected, first of all, with their inhibiting influence on antigen-sensitive, not antibody-producing elements. These authors believe the inhibition of immune response may be connected with direct injury to these elements.

It is of interest that the inductive phase of the immune reaction, the phase most sensitive to the immunodepressive effect of steroid hormones, is at the same time in greatest need of physiological concentrations of these hormones for normal development. Adding hydrocortisone to the nutrient medium of the lymph node tissue culture during the productive phase is without effect, whereas during the induction period the hormone in physiological concentrations stimulates, and in higher concentrations inhibits, the synthesis of antibodies (Ambrose 1970; Halliday and Garvey 1964a,b).

In the intact animal, however, administering the hormones in large enough doses can inhibit the humoral immune response in the productive phase (Meshalova 1958; Shemerovskaya 1974; Ducor and Dietrich 1968; Rose 1959). At the same time corticosteroids do not act on passively administered antibodies, which indicates that the influence of hormones is on the process of immunogenesis, not directly on antibodies (Fischel 1953). In the development of the secondary response the preinductive and inductive phases are also most sensitive to hormones (Shemerovskaya 1974; Fagraens 1952). Thus the influence of exogenous corticosteroids on the development of humoral antibodies is rather complex; the character and intensity of this influence depend on many factors.

Evaluating the effects of hormones on the functions of the immune system on the basis of changes in the humoral immune reaction gives some idea of the effect hormones have on the final results of the activity of the system. However, in regard to the mechanisms of this influence, it is important to investigate the influence of corticosteroids on cellular and subcellular levels.

According to present concepts, four basic populations of cells take part in achieving an immune response: stem hematopoietic cells, T- and B-lymphocytes, and macrophages (Fridenshteyn and Chertkov 1969; Bernett 1971; Miller 1975; Unanue 1975). It has been established that ACTH and glucocorticoids administered to the organism in large enough doses can change the structure and functions of all these elements. The lymphotropic effect of corticosteroids is well known. Reports in the literature include lymphcytolysis, pycnosis of nuclei, and karyorrhexis, which developed several hours after a single administration of corticosteroids. The greatest changes were observed in the thymus and in germinal centers of the spleen and lymph nodes (Zak et al. 1975; Dougherty et al. 1960, 1964; Dougherty and White 1947; Lance and Cooper 1970). Only hormones of the glucocorticoid group have such an effect; the mineralocorticoids do not cause destructive changes in lymphocytes (Dougherty et al. 1964; Dougherty and Schneebeli 1955). The effect of glucocorticoids is observed not only in vivo but also in vitro (Dougherty 1953; Dougherty et al. 1964). Steroid hormones decrease the number of lymphocytes circulating in the blood (Bilenko et al. 1975; Dougherty and White 1947). Inhibition of mitotic cell division is one of the manifestations of the effect of glucocorticoids and ACTH (Laguchev 1975; Dougherty et al. 1964; Eives et al. 1964; Hansen 1957; Ishidate and Metcalf 1963; Tormey et al. 1967). The glucocorticoids inhibit the transformation of lymphocytes under the influence of mitogenic stimuli (Balow et al. 1975; Eives et al. 1964; Tormey et al. 1967). However, according to other data these hormones have a weak influence on the percentage of cells transformed (Darzynkiewicz and Pienkowski 1969).

ACTH and glucocorticoids can suppress the migration capabilities of lymphocytes of peripheral lymph nodes, spleen, and thymus (Petrov et al. 1975; Shannon and Jones 1974). The intensity of the influence of glucocorticoids on lymphocytes, as well as their influ-

ence on humoral immune reactions, depends on the hormone dosages used. Marked structural and functional changes in lymphoid tissue are usually caused by large doses (Mikhaylova 1953; Balow et al. 1975; Dougherty et al. 1964; Hilgar 1968). However, other authors reported effects of relatively small doses of glucocorticoids on this process. Thus Tormey et al. (1967) observed an inhibition of transformation and mitoses of lymphocytes in response to phytohemagglutinin at concentrations of prednisolone in the tissue culture equal to 0.03 $\mu g/ml$.

As many authors have reported, large doses of corticosteroids have marked inhibitory effects on antibody-forming cells (Yekhneva 1975; Uteshev and Babichev 1974; Craddock et al. 1967a,b). Cortisol depressed the plasmocyte reaction in rabbit lymph nodes caused by antigen, while desoxycorticosterone increased it (Gurvich 1963; Zdrodovskiy 1969). In experiments by Chebotarev (1966), hydrocortisone had the same effect. However, Yurina et al. (1975) noted an increase in the number of plasma cells in lymph nodes and bone marrow in immunized and nonimmunized animals under the influence of glucocorticoids. Desoxycorticosterone acetate produced similar changes.

According to some reports, ACTH and glucocorticoids can have an influence on stem cells of the bone marrow. Large doses of hydrocortisone (40 mg/kg) caused depression of the stem elements (Floerscheim 1970). Administering ACTH to mice in a dose of 1.5 units and hydrocortisone in a dose of 20 mg/kg markedly inhibited the migration of stem cells from the bone marrow, T-lymphocytes from the thymus, and B-lymphocytes from the bone marrow in experiments by Petrov et al. (1975). The authors believe this effect can play an essential role in the regulating influence of the hypophysial adrenal system on antibody development.

At the same time it was found that hydrocortisone in a dosage of 125 mg/kg stimulates interaction between polypotent stem hematopoietic cells and cells of the thymus in mice, intensifying the proliferative activity of the former in experiments with cell transfer in irradiated recipients; a dosage of 20 mg/kg was ineffective (Kozlov and Tsyrlova 1975). In vitro experiments revealed no significant decreases in the number of stem cells in mice under the influence of hydrocortisone administered in doses of 1–2 mg four times a day for 4

days (Bennett and Cudkowich 1968). The formation of colonies of bone marrow cells in tissue culture was also inhibited only in response to large doses of cortisone (Metcalf 1969).

The cells of the macrophage series are also subject to the influence of glucocorticoids, but the data on the character of this influence are contradictory. Some investigators found intensified phagocytic activity of macrophages under the influence of hormones (Dougherty and Schneebeli 1950; Luria et al. 1951; Snell 1960); others reported a decrease in phagocytosis as well as in digesting activity of the macrophages (Meshalova 1961; Meshalova and Fryazinova 1960; Fialkow et al. 1973; Kinnaert et al. 1972; Nicol and Belbey 1960; Sloneker and Lim 1972); and some authors found no effects of hormones on the cells (Hirsch and Church 1961; Northe 1971). Wahl et al. (1975) did not observe changes in the migration capability of macrophages under the influence of various doses of glucocorticoids. It was established that the influence of cortisone on macrophage functions (in particular, on the aggregation capability) depends on hormone dosages (Gaumer et al. 1974).

According to most authors, who take into account the time of hormone administration in relation to the time of immunization, it is most effective to give hormones during the first few days before adminstering antigen or during the first few hours or days after immunization (Uteshev and Babichev 1974; Craddock et al. 1967b). However, in some investigations different time relations were observed. Thus Bernasconi et al. (1967) detected a decrease in the number of antibody-forming cells in mice following administration of prednisolone only during the productive phase, from the 3d to the 8th day after immunization with sheep erythrocytes.

For an understanding of the mechanism of the effects of corticosteroids on the immune response in the intact organism, apparently of great significance is the phenomenon, reported by many investigators, of differing hormone sensitivities of lymphoid cells with different characteristics. Lymphocytes of mice, rats, and rabbits are more sensitive to glucocorticoids than are the lymphocytes of guinea pigs, monkeys, and humans (Claman 1975; Rose 1959; Schwell and Long 1956). Long-living lymphocytes are more resistant to the effects of hormones than are short-living ones (Esteban 1968; Miller and Cole 1967). Lymphocytes of the thymus are more sensitive to

the action of glucocorticoids than are cells of the spleen and lymph nodes (Dougherty et al. 1964). Zak et al. (1975) observed opposite changes in various populations of lymphocytes under the influence of hydrocortisone: in the lymphocytes of the thymus, appendix, thymus-dependent zones of lymph nodes, and spleen, they observed atrophy and pycnosis. In other lymphocyte populations they observed changes indicating an increase in cell functions. It was established that lymphocytes of blood of thymus origin suffer more from the administration of glucocorticoids than do B-cells (Fanci 1975).

In very convincing experiments with transfer of corticosteroid-resistant cells into lethally irradiated recipients that were not capable of producing antibodies, it was established that cells resistant to hormonal effects participate in the humoral immune response and can even cause a more intense immune process than can normal cells. As shown in mice (Levine and Claman 1970; Weston et al. 1973), 12.5 mg of cortisone acetate administered 48 and 12 hours before sacrificing the donor animals has completely different effects on the cells of the spleen than on bone marrow cells. Transferring these cells (only of spleen or bone marrow in the presence of thymus cells) into the organism of an irradiated recipient together with sheep erythrocytes sharply lowered the capability of the spleen cells to produce antibodies, whereas the bone marrow cells retained this capability. Cortisone removed the response of spleen cells to phytohemagglutinin but raised this response in bone marrow cells. The authors think that the different inhibiting effect of cortisone may reflect the presence of thymus-dependent cortisone-sensitive cells in the spleen, while the cells of the bone marrow are cortisone resistant and probably thymus independent. In other experiments it was established that cortisone-resistant cells of the thymus, while themselves not capable of producing antibodies (they did not give a humoral response in lethally irradiated recipients), cause at the same time, in comparison with cells of the normal thymus, a raised antibody production in thymectomized lethally irradiated animals with restored bone marrow. No drop in the immune capability of resistant cells of the spleen was noted, even though the dosage of cortisone acetate was 125 mg/kg (Andersson and Blomgren 1970). The preservation of capability to participate in humoral responses of cortisone-resistant cells

of the thymus has been confirmed by Andersson and Blomgren (1971) and J. J. Cohen (1971).

As experiments by E. P. Cohen et al. (1970) have shown, the glucocorticoids decrease the number of cells in the thymus, spleen, and bone marrow. However, the number of hormone-resistant cells that remain in these structures following administration of 2.5 mg of cortisone to mice 2 days before transfer differs: in thymus 6%, in spleen 21%, in bone marrow 79%. The remaining cells, upon transfer to neonatal recipients, retain their capability for cell immune reactions; they cause more actively than do the cells of control animals the "transplant against host" reaction. Similar data were obtained by Kozlov et al. (1974).

The corticosteroid-resistant cells of the thymus retain the ability of rosella formation (Bach and Dardenne 1971) and proliferation (Blomgren 1971). They increase synthesis of DNA in response to antigen stimulation (Cohen and Gershon 1975) and retain the capability of blast transformation under the influence of phytohemagglutinin. Adding glucocorticoids in large doses to cortisone-resistant thymocytes in vitro suppresses the synthesis of protein in these cells, but less than in the controls (Weissman and Levy 1975). Thus corticosteroid-resistant lymphocytes can retain the capability of humoral as well as cellular immune response.

From these data it follows that the decrease in the number of cells in individual lymphoid tissues, or changes in their functions and structures, observed by many authors cannot always be interpreted as indicating inhibition of immune capabilities of the lymphoid system in the intact organism.

The biochemical basis for the influence of steroid hormones on structures and functions of lymphoid cells consists in their effect on various metabolic changes. Detailed data on these mechanisms are given in surveys by Sergeyev et al. (1971) and Eisenstein (1973). Sergeyev et al. (1971) considered several aspects of the action of steroid hormones on cells of the immunocompetent system:

1. Interaction of the hormone with membrane structures that is the result of a definite connection of the physicochemical properties of the steroid molecule with receptors of cell membranes.

2. Penetration of the steroid molecule through the changed plas-

ma membrane into the cell where binding of the hormone with specific cytoplasmic receptor proteins takes place.

3. Penetration of the steroid into the cell nucleus and the interaction with repressor proteins, so that definite sections of the cell genome
are repressed.

4. Secondary changes in the permeability of cell membranes as a
result of de novo synthesis of ribonucleic acids and specific enzyme
molecules as well as changes in the topography of enzyme actions.

The process of binding glucocorticoids with receptor proteins of
lymphocytes is apparently the first reaction of their interaction.
Physicochemical principles of binding hormones by receptor molecules are described in detail in a survey by Rozen (1973). The presence of receptors to glucocorticoids in lymphoid cells has been established in a number of investigations. The intensity of binding
hormones is proportional to the biological activity of the hormones;
they do not interact with inactive metabolites of glucocorticoids
(Rozen 1973).

It is of great interest that the receptors to glucocorticoids were
found in cells of structures taking part in the regulation of the functions of the hypothalamohypophysio-adrenocortical system (HHAS),
including the amygdala and hippocampus. The physiological role of
cytoreceptors and the complexing of steroid hormones with cell proteins apparently consists first of all in the capture and accumulation
of hormones by target cells from the tissue fluids. The complexing
of hormones facilitates their penetration into the cell, apparently
against a concentration gradient. The same processes can, in the
opinion of Rozen (1973), play a definite role in the regulation by
hormones of biosynthesis of ribonucleic acids. However, the question of the physiological role of hormone receptors in general and
receptors of lymphoid cells in particular requires further study.

One of the most investigated molecular mechanisms involved in
the effects of steroid hormones on lymphoid system cells is the reduction in protein synthesis in lymphoid tissues. This effect has been
well demonstrated in experiments in which a considerable lowering
was observed in the inclusion of marked amino acids in the general
cell proteins and protein fractions of the thymus, spleen, and lymph
nodes under the influence of ACTH or glucocorticoids. Administering glucocorticoids causes marked inhibition of the inclusion of

marked amino acids into DNA and a reduction in its total content in individual lymphoid tissues; it also inhibits DNA synthesis.

Analysis of literature data on the mechanism of the effect of glucocorticoids on lymphoid tissue permitted Sergeyev et al. (1971) to come to a conclusion concerning the primary interaction of hormones with the repressor system. This interaction leads to a change in its metabolism, lowering the matrix of DNA activity. However, the question of the mechanisms by which steroids interact with immunocompetent cells in the intact organism remains unclear. It must be emphasized that in most of the reports dealing with the influence of hormones on various aspects of protein synthesis in lymphoid tissues, very large doses of hormones were used. Where the influence of hormones in a definite range of doses was investigated, the inhibiting effect of hormones on protein synthesis was dose dependent (Gabourel and Comstock 1964; Stevens et al. 1965). Unfortunately, even in these experiments, as a rule, the hormone dosages used were far from those encountered under physiological conditions. Therefore one can form only approximate conclusions on the role of glucocorticoids in protein metabolism of lymphoid cells under physiological conditions.

Ambrose (1970) proposed an interesting hypothesis on the influence of glucocorticoids on protein metabolism in lymphoid cells. According to his data, hydrocortisone added to rabbit lymph node tissue cultures in physiological concentrations facilitates the stimulating effect of small doses of actinomycin D on the synthesis of antibodies as well as the inhibitory effect of large doses of this preparation on the immune process during the productive phase when the hydrocortisone itself was not necessary for the development of an immune reaction. The author suggests that the permissive effect of the hormone is due to its demasking effect on DNA chromatin, which makes the molecules accessible to the influence of various stimuli.

One of the possible mechanisms of the influence of hormones (including ACTH and glucocorticoids) on immunocompetent cells is their ability to change the metabolism of cyclic nucleotides: adenosine-3',5'-cyclomonophosphate and guanosine-3',5'-cyclomonophosphate. The bases for this assumption were, on the one hand, data on the influence of hormones on the activity of cyclic nucleo-

tides in immunocompetent cells (Claman 1975; Haolden 1975; Kemp and Dugueskoy 1975; Schmutzler and Freundt 1975) and, on the other hand, changes in the activity of cyclomonophosphates and guanomonophosphates during immunization (Braun 1973; Park et al. 1974; Plescia et al. 1975; Uzonova 1974) and the effect of exogenous cyclic nucleotides on the immune response (Bösing-Scheider 1975; Braun and Ishizuka 1971; Ishizuka et al. 1971; Mednieks and Danute 1975; Ten and Paetkau 1974). Of significance is the influence of hormones on the sensitivity of cyclic nucleotides to mediators (Kemp and Dugueskoy 1975; Kemp et al. 1973; Queiroz et al. 1975; Schmutzler and Freundt 1975).

In concluding the survey of studies dealing with the influence of exogenous hormones of the hypophyseal-adrenocortical system on immune processes, certain characteristic features of this influence must be emphasized. From these data it follows that exogenous ACTH and glucocorticoids administered to the intact organism exert marked influence on the functions of the immune system, manifested in changes in the structure of the cells taking part in immune reactions and changes in their biochemical status, proliferative capacities, migration processes, and capacity to produce antibodies.

It is important to emphasize that the character and intensity of the influence of these hormones on the humoral immune response, as well as on the structure and functions of cells of the lymphoid system, depend both on the dosages of the hormone and on the dosages and immunogenic properties of antigen used. Small doses of corticosteroids, approximating physiological range, are apparently essential for the normal course of immune reactions and normal functioning of lymphoid cells. Higher dosages of hormones exert immunodepressive effects, which manifest themselves in decreases in humoral immune reactions, inhibition of division in mitotic cells, and even cell destruction. It should be emphasized that the humoral immune reactions produced by sufficiently strong antigens cannot easily be inhibited by hormones. To substantially depress humoral immune reactions in such a system, the dose of the hormone and its period of application must be considerably increased.

At the same time, as follows from the data described above, the changes in the functions of lymphoid cells and their number of individual immunocompetent tissues were often observed after adminis-

tration of single moderate doses of corticosteroids. This contradiction, it seems to us, can be explained by the marked difference in sensitivity to corticosteroids of various lymphoid elements, demonstrated by convincing experiments. Inasmuch as the corticosteroid-resistant lymphocytes are immunocompetent, it is possible to hypothesize that, following certain doses of hormones administered to the organism, changes can be observed in a number of cells, and in their structure and functions in individual lymphoid populations, without noticeable change in the humoral immune reaction of the entire system, which occurs at the expense of the activity of elements resistant to hormones. However, it is not known to what extent and in what range of hormonal doses the capabilities of cells resistant to antibody production appear. As experimental data suggest, prolonged administration of large doses of corticosteroids always lowers antibody formation, though with administration of a high enough dose of strong antigen, the corticosteroids are not capable of completely inhibiting the development of humoral antibodies (Darrach 1959).

In evaluating the influence of corticosteroids on immune reactions in the intact organism, these hormones should not be considered only as immunodepressants. Immunodepressive effects in the intact organism can appear only in response to appropriate dosages of the hormones administered and level of intensity of the antigen-produced process, and in relation to only a definite fraction of the cells of the immunocompetent system.

Data obtained after administration of exogenous hormones also furnish the basis for understanding the links of the immune process most sensitive to hormones. As was demonstrated above, on the one hand, the induction phase of the immune reaction needs physiological concentrations of corticosteroids, and on the other hand, it is most sensitive to the inhibitory influence of high doses of hormones. To obtain an inhibitory effect, the presence of hormones in the blood at the moment of immunization is not obligatory; it is important that hormonal actions on the cells have occurred several hours before the antigen is administered. The period of semidecomposition of glucocorticoids in the organism must not exceed 1.5–4 hours (Komissarenko and Reznikov 1972; Klegg and Klegg 1971). At the same time, hormones administered to the organism 24 and 48 hours

before immunization may have some influence on the immune response. These data confirm that glucocorticoids apparently cause the most perceptible changes at the level of antigen-sensitive elements. However, this does not mean that corticosteroids in general cannot exert influences during later stages of the immune process. Probably, at sufficiently large doses, they can also inhibit the antibody-producing cells, since a number of authors have obtained data on the effect of hormones administered during the productive phase.

Apparently the biochemical basis for the influence of corticosteroids on immune processes is, first of all, their kinetic interaction with protein structures of immunocompetent cells and their influence on protein metabolism. It must be noted that studies were conducted primarily on the influence of high doses of hormones, and it has been established that they cause a reduction in protein synthesis in lymphoid tissues. Indeed, this mechanism explains well the inhibition of mitotic cell division and the decrease of antibody synthesis in response to high doses of exogenous hormones. However, this mechanism does not explain why the corticosteroids are necessary in physiological concentrations for the development of a normal immune reaction, or why small doses of these hormones can stimulate a humoral response or the functions of macrophages. It is also not known what happens with protein metabolism of cortisone-resistant cells after exogenous administration of high doses of hormones. Taking into account that the immune capabilities of these cells do not decrease, and sometimes even increase, one may assume that the corticosteroids do not depress protein metabolism of these cell elements. Of great interest also is the cyclomonophosphate of these cells, inasmuch as its considerable role has been shown in the process of antibody synthesis.

Examining the influence of exogenous hormones of the hypophysio-adrenocortical system in the intact organism, one must take into account the possibility that they have a mediating effect on immunocompetent structures. Such mechanisms of the action of exogenous hormones exist, and here, first of all, one must consider the role of the CNS, which actively participates in the regulation of the synthesis and release of hormones and in the sensitivity of tissues to their actions (Aleshin 1971; Komissarenko and Reznikov 1972; Lissak and Endröczi 1967). One must take into account the liver, which plays an important role in the utilizing of hormones and in the in-

hibitory effects of hormones on synthetic processes in lymphoid tissues (Sergeyev et al. 1971).

Endogenous Hormones of the Hypophysio-adrenocortical System and Immune Reactions

Data on the influence of endogenous hormones of the hypophysio-adrenocortical system on immune reactions have added essentially to our concepts of possible hormonal regulation of immune reactions in the organism. In clinical medicine hormonal preparations of the glucocorticoid group are widely used to depress immune reactions, together with other immunodepressants. However, for developing concepts of neuroendocrine regulation of the immune process in the organism, these data are insufficient. The problem is that, as mentioned before, most researchers have used dosages of hormones specifically designed to inhibit immune reactions. Only a few have studied dose-effect relationships. To discover the mechanisms of interactions of the neuroendocrine and immune systems in achieving reactions of specific protection, it is important to establish first of all what influence the physiological shifts in the concentration of endogenous hormones have on the immune process under conditions of increased or decreased functioning of the HHAS. No less important are investigations of those hormonal shifts that accompany the development of a normal or pathologically changed immune reaction and correlations between immunologic and hormonal indexes.

As we know, the most common state of the organism involving the stimulating effect of the adrenopituitary system is stress (Selye 1952, 1972). Studies of the influence of stress on immune reactions have produced inconsistent results. On the one hand, certain types of stress apparently do not essentially influence the humoral immune response. In experiments with mice subjected for 2–15 days before and after immunization to an electric current, no changes were observed in the number of neutralizing antibodies in serum in response to the virus of vesicular stomatitis (Yamada et al. 1964). Solomon (1969b) did not observe essential changes in immune reactions to the flagelline polymer obtained from *Salmonella adelaide* in rats subjected to low-voltage electrical stimulation through the paws five times in one hour in the course of a week before immunization and

the entire subsequent period of observation. On the other hand, a strong light or sound stress inhibited the formation of antibodies in response to ox albumin in monkeys (Hill et al. 1967). A lowering of the primary and secondary immune response to the flagelline polymer from *Salmonella adelaide* in rats was reported (Solomon 1969b), as well as the primary response to ox serum in mice (Vessey 1964), under conditions of crowding in the animals' cages.

Effects of stress on immune reactions were reported by Zdrodovskiy and Gurvich (1972). Various types of stress in experiments conducted by these authors reproduced anamnestic serologic reactions and activated the production of specific globulins in previously immunized rats. In the opinion of Solomon (1969b), acute stress, even if applied frequently, does not activate immunodepressive mechanisms, presumably because applying stressors for short periods permits the organism to adapt to them. Only chronic types of stress (which lead to prolonged reactions that extinguish poorly) are immunodepressive.

However, there are data in the literature showing that even a single application of a stressor can change the immune reactivity of lymphoid cells. The application of a single stressor (rotation in a centrifuge, ether narcosis) significantly inhibits immune reactivity of spleen cells cultured in vitro with sheep erythrocytes. The stress proved immunodepressive if the stressors were applied 6, 16, or 24 hours before immunization. However, cells removed from the donor 15 minutes after the stressor was applied gave definite results. The inhibitory effect of stressors on the cells of the spleen correlated with the increased content of corticosterone in the blood caused by the applied stimuli. Seventy-five hours after exposure to the stressor (when the content of corticosterone had decreased) the immunodepressive effect was not observed. A single administration of ACTH reproduced the stressor effects during the period of maximal corticosterone in the blood; in adrenalectomized animals, the preparation had no effect. In hypophysectomized mice, a marked suppression of immune reactivity of spleen cells was observed (Gisler et al. 1971; Gisler and Schenkel-Hullinger 1971). Electric shock applied for 7 days can decrease the reactivity of cells of the lymph nodes and spleen to concanavalin A and phytohemagglutinin (Solomon et al. 1974). In the same study, an inhibition of "transplant against host" reaction was shown in recipients subjected to partial

starvation for 7 days before injection of donor lymphocytes as well as later in the development of the immune reaction. At the same time, lymphocytes from a donor subjected to stress were fully capable of causing a normal reaction. Therefore the authors concluded that the effect of stress occurs not as a result of injury to the lymphoid population of the donor, but from changes in the processes of interaction between the cells in the recipient organism, or processes of release of mediators by the reacting lymphocytes.

It is of interest that the lowering of the number of circulating lymphocytes caused by a 24 hour exposure to a stressor applied immediately after administration of poliomyelitis virus to monkeys was correlated with a marked rise in resistance in these animals (March et al. 1963).

In evaluating the data above, one should take into account that changes in cell reactivity of certain parts of the lymphoid system apparently cannot fully reflect the activity of the immune system in the intact organism, which might explain some of the contradictions in the data obtained in the study of the influence of stress on humoral and cellular reactions. Zdrodovskiy (1969) described a directly opposite effect of cold stress on the plasmocyte reaction in the regional lymph nodes and agglutinins in the blood. Stressors inhibited plasmocytosis and lowered agglutinin titers in regional lymph nodes in rats previously twice immunized with the full antigen of Gärtner bacillus; but they led to a rise in the titers of agglutinins in the blood, corresponding in time to a decrease in the titers and plasmocytes in the lymph nodes. All these changes occurred during the first 3 days of the stress effect, that is, during the "anxiety reaction" (Selye 1960), after which the indicators returned to normal. In the opinion of Zdrodovskiy (Zdrodovskiy 1962, 1969, 1971; Zdrodovskiy and Gurvich 1972), an increase in the titers of antibodies in the blood can be the result of their passive introduction under the influence of stress-induced release of corticosteroids. However, it is possible that this is not the only explanation, inasmuch as the blood antibody content may depend on the activity of all immunocompetent cells in the entire immune system, whereas the sensitivity to hormones of different populations of lymphocytes may not be identical.

Apparently, in the effect of stressors as well as in the effect of the influence of exogenous hormones on immune reactions, the intensity of the hormonal shift caused by the applied stimulus, the time of

its application relative to the administration of antigen, and the properties and dosages of the antigen all play definite roles. The duration of the stress also plays a role, since adaptation to it proceeds in several stages, differing in their physiological and biochemical characteristics (Selye 1960, 1972). Moreover, it should not be forgotten that stress is a state of the organism to which are natural not only an increase in the levels of ACTH and glucocorticoids, but also more complex neuroendocrine shifts, including changes in the level of mineralocorticoids (Selye 1960, 1972); somatotropin (Brown and Reichlin 1972; Dunn et al. 1973–74; Franchimont et al. 1970; McIntyre and Odell 1974; Meites et al. 1974); thyrotrophin and hormones of the thyroid gland (Zaychik 1971; Zenzerov et al. 1973; Pel'ts 1955; Eastman et al. 1974; Jong and Moll 1965); sex hormones (Krulich et al. 1974; Meites et al. 1974); and biogenic amines (Aleshin 1971; Selye 1960; Shreiber 1963).

The intensity of changes in the concentration of hormones and mediators, and their interaction, apparently depends on the intensity of the stimulus and its character, which in turn can determine the direction and intensity of the influences of various stressors on the immmune reaction. Inasmuch as the individual components of this humoral complex may have opposing effects on immune processes, the results of stress will apparently depend not only on each of them separately, but also on their general interaction.

In some studies of recent years, attempts were made to discover how the function of the immune system relates to diurnal rhythms of hormone content. Shargin and Povazhenko (1974) established that the correlation of T- and B-rosella-forming cells in the course of a day is not constant in humans: T-rosella-forming cells were at a maximum in the morning hours, B-rosella-forming cells in the evening. The authors relate these differences to diurnal fluctuations in plasma 11-hydroxycorticosteroids. The level of serum agglutinins in mice is twice as high in the evening as in the daytime (Fernandes et al. 1974). Since in mice the content of glucocorticoids rises precisely in the evening, there is no basis for thinking that the observed differences are due to the immunodepressive effect of these hormones. Apparently the origin of diurnal variations of immune indexes is more complex.

Additional data on the mechanism of the effects of endogenous

corticosteroids on immune reactions could be obtained from experiments with selective exclusion of the adrenocorticotropic function of the hypophysis or the glucocorticoid function of the adrenal cortex. However, such a selective exclusion is very difficult to achieve. One of the methods that could be used for this purpose is the administration of antiadrenocorticotropic serum. But since such serum of sufficiently high titer is very difficult to procure, in connection with a comparatively small molecular weight of the hormones (Fedotov and Sokolov 1970), until recently the investigations were limited basically to the influence of surgical removal of the hypophysis or the adrenals.

There are many reasons why evaluating data on such experiments is difficult. First of all, as a rule removing glands causes complex disturbances of hormonal balance: factors may be excluded that affect the immune reactions in an opposite direction. For example, removing the adrenal cortex excludes not only the glucocorticoids but also the mineralocorticoids, whose activities with respect to the immune process, as was shown above, are quite different. Removing the entire adrenal gland, which is most often done, leads to still more complex effects, inasmuch as the catecholamine balance (which plays an important role in the development of immune reactions) is disturbed (Kozlov 1968; Marat 1973, 1975; Frolov 1974). An even more complex hormonal shift occurs upon removal of the hypophysis, the endocrine organ generating hormones whose effect on immune reactions under different conditions can have opposite effects (somatotropin, adrenocorticotropin, thyrotropin). Sometimes removing the gland does not completely exclude its function, since additional endocrine formations exist in many animals. Moreover, in these types of experiments, different substitution therapies were used as well as different types and dosages of antigens. As was shown in detail above, the properties and dosages of antigens play an important role in the changes corticosteroid hormones cause in the immune process. These factors may explain the contradictory results often obtained in such experiments.

In some experiments adrenalectomy intensified humoral immune reactions and stimulated cell reactions (Kopytovskaya 1970; Yarilin and Polushkina 1975; Char and Kelley 1962; Criep et al. 1951; Streng and Nathan 1973); in other experiments it led to inhibition

(Ivanov 1963, 1964; Chebotarev and Valuyeva 1972; Benetato et al. 1958; Roberts and White 1951); and finally, some authors did not observe any changes after such surgical procedures (Dews and Code 1953; Thatcher et al. 1948). Petrov et al. (1975) found in adrenalectomized mice a marked increase in the migration of hematopoietic stem cells from the bone marrow, which caused the content of these cells in the peripheral blood and spleen to increase markedly. Excluding the function of the adrenal glands by administering antiadrenal serum decreased the number of antibody-forming cells in the spleen in response to immunization with sheep erythrocytes in experiments by Zdrodovskiy and Gurvich (1972). The immune response could be stimulated by administering desoxycorticosterone or somatotropin.

No less contradictory results were obtained in experiments with the exclusion of the hypophysis. According to many data (Kalden et al. 1970; Molomut 1939; Thrasher et al. 1971; Tyrey and Nalbandov 1972), hypophysectomy does not cause essential changes in the course of immune reactions. However, Pierpaoli and Sorkin (1969a,b) found that administering antihypophyseal serum to young sexually active mice considerably lowers immune reactivity, according to cellular and humoral indicators. Similar data were obtained by Zdrodovskiy and Gurvich (1972). Administering antihypophyseal serum in these experiments decreased the number of antibody-forming cells in rat spleen as a response to sheep erythrocytes.

As Lundin (1960) showed, hypophysectomy lowers the immune response in rats only if small threshold doses of antigen are given; it also causes in rats a disturbance in the restoration of the total number of leukocytes and the humoral immune response to sheep erythrocytes after subtotal irradiation (Dugueskoy et al. 1969).

The influence of the hypophysis on the immune system is most clearly shown during early ontogenesis. In a series of experiments on hypophyseal dwarf mice, hypotrophy of the thymus and peripheral lymphoid tissue was observed as well as a marked inhibition of antibody formation (Baroni et al. 1967; Dugueskoy et al. 1969; Pierpaoli et al. 1969; Pierpaoli and Sorkin 1967, 1969b; Sorkin and Pierpaoli 1970).

The authors conclude that the development of lymphatic tissue in the neonatal and perinatal periods in mice depends on the hypophysis. As we will show later, inhibition of the development of the thymus

and lymphoid tissue in mice with congenital underdeveloped hypophyses is related chiefly to insufficiency of somatotropin and thyrotropin. It is not known whether decrease in ACTH function has any role in these animals, since no experiments have been conducted with anti-ACTH serum.

In the adult organism, the interrelations of the hypophysis and lymphoid tissue are not as clear. Probably, to achieve comparable results after hypophysectomy, the following must be strictly controlled: the species and age of the animals, type and dosages of antigen, and time of immunization relative to hypophysectomy.

As follows from the above, the results obtained in experiments with hypophysectomy or adrenalectomy do not make it possible to determine definitively what role endogenous hormones of the hypophysio-adrenal system play in the development of an immune reaction in the organism. Therefore, to elucidate this, it is important to directly measure the level of hormones in the blood and tissues during various phases of the immune process in intact animals as well as in animals with extirpated endocrine glands.

There are few investigations of this kind. Until recently researchers primarily studied the hormonal shifts accompanying the process of sensitization or characterizing various forms of already formed hypersensitive states. Since the immunologic and biochemical mechanisms of these states are very complex, the data on hormonal shifts are difficult to analyze. Yet to understand the character and the mechanisms of origin of changes in HHAS function during formation of an immune reaction, it is necessary to answer the following questions:

1. What is the character of the changes in the function of the HHAS during the various phases of development of an immune process in the organism under normal conditions?

2. What mechanisms participate in producing hormonal shifts accompanying the development of an immune reaction?

3. How does the functional state of the HHAS change under conditions of inhibition or stimulation of the immune process?

4. Is there a correlation between hormonal shifts and the intensity of immune reactions in different phases of an immune reaction?

To answer these questions, we conducted experiments with direct measurement of the level of glucocorticoids in blood plasma and of immune indicators in serum during the development of primary im-

mune reactions in rabbits and mice. Glucocorticoid concentrations were measured on the basis of total 11-hydroxycorticosteroids (Pankov and Usvatova 1965). The level of antibodies was measured according to the reaction of complement binding (Ioffe and Rozental' 1943), reactions of agglutination (Vyazov and Khodzhayeva 1973), or passive hemagglutination (Kraskina and Gutorova 1962). As antigen we used, in the experiments with rabbits, normal warmed horse serum in a dosage of 0.25 ml/kg and Vi-antigen of typhoid bacillus in a dosage of 8 μg/kg (produced by the Moscow Institute of Microbiology and Epidemiology). In the experiments with mice we used rat erythrocytes in a dosage of 2×10^7 and sheep erythrocytes in a dosage of 2×10^9 per animal. All antigens were injected intravenously.

We established that a single immunization causes a regular rise in the concentration of total 11-OH-CS in the plasma in the first hours after introduction of the antigens (Shkhinek et al. 1974). Horse serum led to an increase in the level of 11-OH-CS within 20–30 minutes; the reaction reached a maximum in some animals at 12 hours, in others, at 2–4 hours after immunization. The reaction to the typhoid bacillus Vi-antigen developed still faster: its maximum in all animals occurred 1–2 hours after immunization; after 24 hours the level of hormones decreased (table 5). The intensity of the hormonal shift in response to these antigens was on the average 45–65% with respect to the initial level. Still greater changes in the concentration of hormones were observed in mice in response to the administration of heterologous erythrocytes: the level of 11-OH-CS 1–2 hours after immunization, at the height of the reaction, was 150% of the control; by 4 hours the level had decreased considerably, and in 24 hours it had returned to normal. During the first few days, no antibodies could be detected in any of these cases (figs. 27 and 35, curve 1).

Thus, the inductive phase of the development of an immune reaction is characterized by a rise in concentration of glucocorticoid hormones in the blood. Similar data were obtained by Belovolova (1973), who immunized rabbits with fraction I of plague microbe. The maximum of the reaction in these experiments was observed 1–3 hours after immunization, and the intensity of the shift was approximately 100–200%.

In investigating humoral changes in the dynamics of the further development of immune reactions, we found no regular shifts. In a

Table 5   Changes in Concentration of 11-Hydroxycorticosteroids in Blood Plasma (μg/100 ml) in the Course of the First Days after Immunization in Rabbits

Numbers of Groups and Statistical Indicators	Time after Immunization (hours)											
	Immunization with Horse Serum				Immunization with Vi-Antigen of Typhoid Bacillus				Administration of Physiological Solution			
	0	1	2	24	0	1	2	24	0	1	2	24
1	3.6	4.3	4.2	—	6.1	9.3	11.6	8.9	8.1	7.5	4.7	—
2	2.8	3.0	4.6	5.0	5.0	7.5	6.5	6.9	10.3	6.4	7.4	—
3	8.9	—	14.5	13.3	5.8	6.6	12.1	9.5	10.9	7.5	7.5	—
4	10.4	—	16.4	14.8	6.0	7.8	10.1	7.2	8.0	6.6	6.9	7.6
5	4.3	8.6	6.6	7.9	6.7	7.8	10.1	7.5	8.2	5.9	8.1	7.1
6	3.4	8.8	6.8	5.2	4.2	8.5	4.6	4.1	4.9	4.9	—	5.9
7	4.7	8.2	7.8	6.8	2.5	9.1	4.6	3.6	6.8	6.2	7.3	7.1
8	2.5	—	1.3	1.5	5.5	3.8	6.9	5.4	4.4	3.4	4.4	3.9
9	10.4	11.1	14.4	12.0	6.0	10.6	12.0	8.0	7.9	4.2	4.2	4.2
10	10.4	—	8.4	6.4	3.8	6.8	8.0	3.6	2.3	1.5	—	—
11	10.4	11.0	12.8	6.7	2.5	6.4	3.8	3.2	5.7	5.4	4.8	3.2
12					4.6	6.7	7.9	3.4	3.9	4.8	4.5	6.0
13					6.9	9.6	10.0	11.3				
14					7.4	11.0	12.7	6.6				
M	6.2	7.9	8.9	8.0	5.2	7.9	8.6	6.4	6.8	5.4	6.0	5.6
t		0	6.5	16		3	0	16		5.0	7.0	9.0
P		<.01	<.05	>.05		<.01	<.01	<.01		<.01	<.05	>.05

Note: In each of the groups, different animals were used. Processed by the Wilcoxon two-sample t-test (Gubler and Genkin 1973) with respect to the initial level before immunization.

series of experiments with Vi-antigen, the level of hormones in all animals returned to its initial values after 1–2 days, and in the course of the whole following period of investigation it did not differ from control values (fig. 27). Following administration of heterologous erythrocytes to mice, the concentration of 11-OH-CS returned to normal after 24 hours. On the 6th day (during the period of maximal production of antibodies), the level of 11-OH-CS did not differ from the control values (fig. 35, curve 1). In contrast to this, following immunization with horse serum, after an initial normalization of the level of hormones in the blood from the 3d to the 10th day, a second wave of increase in the concentration of hormones was observed on the 14–20th days, that is, during maximal antibody production; this effect was not very marked in all animals (fig. 27).

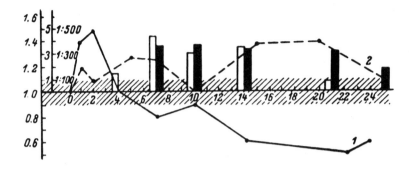

Fig. 27   Dynamics of concentration of 11-hydroxycorticosteroids of plasma
and antibody titers of rabbit serum at various periods of development of immune responses to Vi-antigen of typhoid bacillus (1) and
horse serum (2). *Open bars,* antibody titers in group 1; *solid bars,*
antibody titers in group 2; *striped area,* range of variations of 11-
hydroxycorticosteroids before immunization (confidence interval).
Abscissae, time (days) after immunization; ordinates from left to
right, concentration of 11-hydroxycorticosteroids with respect to
the average level before immunization, taken as 1; titers of complement-binding antibodies (arbitrary units); hemagglutinin titers in
diluted serum.

However, other authors (Belyavskiy 1958; Rozen et al. 1973) found
regular phase changes in the concentration of 11-OH-CS during the
productive stage. In particular, Belovolova (1973) observed a three-
fold rise of 11-OH-CS content in the plasma during formation of the
immune reaction under the influence of fraction I of plague microbe: during the first hours, on the 3d and 10th days after immunization. According to her data, the intensification of the activity of
the HHAS coincided in time with the phase changes of the concentrations of catecholamines and histamine in the blood and tissues of
immunized animals.

It must be noted that a rise in the level of total 11-OH-CS in the
blood during the inductive phase does not fully characterize the
changes in glucocorticoid functions during this period. In particular, the rise in total 11-OH-CS does not make it possible to determine to what extent the levels of physiologically active fractions
have changed.

As is well known from experiments of recent years, glucocorticoids can be found in either a free or a protein-bound state. One of the plasma globulins most actively binding glucocorticoids is corticosteroid-binding globulin or transcortin (see review by Rozen 1973). Some researchers believe that these globulin-binding glucocorticoids serve a transport function, facilitating the transfer of hormones to the cells of target organs. It is possible that the role of transcortin is not limited to this. Since transcortin binds corticosterone in equimolar amounts (Seal and Doe 1962), its concentration in plasma reflects its binding capability. During conjugation with transcortin, the corticosteroids apparently are physiologically inactive (Rozen 1973; Moor et al. 1963; Slaunwhite et al. 1962). Therefore a measure of the intensity of binding of hormones with transcortin, in conjunction with changes of concentration of total 11-OH-CS, could serve as an index not only of total changes in the concentrations of glucocorticoids, but also of their physiological activity. We conducted such an investigation with our colleagues in the Institute of Experimental Medicine of the Hungarian Academy of Sciences (Shkhinek, Ach, and Abavari, unpublished data), utilizing the isotopic method for determining the binding capability of transcortin (Moor 1965) during various periods of the development of the immune process in rabbits. As an antigen we utilized Vi-antigen of typhoid bacillus in a dose of 8 μg/kg. It turned out that in the inductive phase of the immune reaction, in the first hours after immunization, the binding capability of transcortin definitely decreased, and the maximum of this lowering was observed 2 and 24 hours after the administration of antigen (fig. 28), after which the indicators gradually (very slowly) returned to control levels.

Changes in the binding capability of transcortin followed the increase in concentration of total 11-OH-CS in the blood, although there was no perfect correlation (fig. 28). The lowering of the total amount of plasma protein, determined by the method of Lowry (Lowry et al. 1951), was observed in the same period as the drop in the binding capacity of transcortin but later was very quickly restored. The level of antibodies (using the reaction of passive hemagglutination) rose in the period when the content of total 11-OH-CS, the binding capacity of transcortin, and total protein level had almost returned to normal (fig. 28).

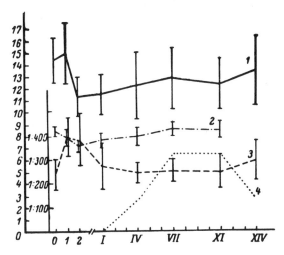

Fig. 28   Changes in the binding power of transcortin (1), total protein (2),
total plasma 11-hydroxycorticosteroids (3), and mean serum hemagglutinin titers (4) in rabbits immunized once with Vi-antigen of
typhoid bacillus. Abscissae, time after immunization (arabic numerals = hours, roman numerals = days); ordinates on the left,
concentration of 11-hydroxycorticosteroids and binding power of
transcortin (μg/100 ml) and concentration of total plasma protein
(g/100 ml); ordinates on the right, antibody titers in diluted serum.
Vertical lines, standard deviations.

These data indicate that the most marked lowering of the binding
capacity of transcortin, as well as the rise in concentration of 11-
OH-CS and the decrease in total proteins, is observed in the inductive phase of the immune response, primarily in the first days after
immunization, when antibodies are still absent from the blood.
Since there is information in the literature on a possible relation between corticosteroid level in plasma and binding capacity of transcortin, it is possible that the changes in binding capability of transcortin we observed are caused by corresponding changes in the
concentration of 11-OH-CS. However, opinions differ concerning
the role of corticosteroids in regulating the binding capability of
transcortin.

According to the data of some authors, the level of transcortin in the blood depends directly on the concentration in the plasma of corticosteroids (Daughaday 1959; Mills et al. 1960), which in rats have an inhibiting effect on the level of transcortin. ACTH administered for several weeks also depresses the binding capacity of transcortin, according to results by Ach et al. (1967); it acts not only by way of the adrenals, since it is also effective in adrenalectomized rats. In the opinion of other authors, the concentration of corticosteroids does not regulate the content of transcortin, at least not in guinea pigs (Yudayev et al. 1966); ACTH is not capable of normalizing the binding capacity of transcortin lowered as a result of hypophysectomy (Antonichev and Rozen 1967). On the basis of these data, researchers conclude that, if the hypophysis does regulate the binding capability of transcortin, then it does so not by means of ACTH but via some other factor (Antonichev and Rozen 1967; Rozen 1973; Rozen et al. 1973; Rozen and Pankova 1971; Yudayev et al. 1966).

According to our data, the lowering of the binding capacity of transcortin did not fully coincide in time with a rise of corticosteroids in plasma. In particular, 1 hour after immunization, when the content of 11-OH-CS in the plasma was maximal, the level of transcortin changed hardly at all (and was even somewhat raised), and after 24 hours when the concentration of 11-OH-CS was returning to the initial level, the level of transcortin was substantially lowered. Data analysis in the following period of the investigation showed a slow normalization of the binding capacity of transcortin. Therefore it is not very likely that the lowered binding capacity of transcortin in our experiments was due to the comparatively temporary rise in concentration of corticosteroids after injection of the antigen.

It is possible that certain properties of the antigen stimulus itself are responsible for the observed effect. In the period of the greatest drop in the binding capacity of transcortin, we also observed a lowering of the concentration of total protein in the plasma. Therefore the possibility that the changes are partially conditioned by a nonspecific influence of immunization on the total protein, found during these periods, is not ruled out. The lowered binding capacity of

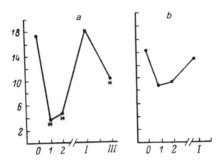

Fig. 29   Changes in aldosterone concentrations in blood plasma of rabbits
                 immunized with sheep erythrocytes (*a*) and Vi-antigen of typhoid
                 bacillus (*b*). Ordinates, concentration of aldosterone (ng/100 ml).
                 Asterisks indicate statistically significant values. Other designa-
                 tions as in figure 28.

transcortin paired with a rise in the general level of 11-OH-CS points
to an increase in the physiologically active fraction of free glucocorticoids in the inductive period of the immune process.

As further experiments showed, the administration of antigen to
the organism can be accompanied by changes in the concentration
not only of glucocorticoids but also of mineralocorticoids. In a series of experiments conducted on rabbits by the radio-immune
method (Shkhinek, Szalai, and Abavari, unpublished data), it was
shown that a single intravenous injection with sheep erythrocytes
causes a drop in aldosterone concentration in the plasma 1 and 2
hours after immunization, utilizing the method of paired Wilcoxon
criteria (Gubler and Genkin 1973), $p < .01$, after which the content
of the hormone rose in 24 hours and by the 3d day dropped again
(fig. 29). Similar changes were observed following immunization
with Vi-antigen of typhoid bacillus; however, in this case the
changes were not statistically significant. It is not known how specific the observed effect is. In some experiments with intravenous injection of a physiological solution, similar changes were observed.
However, there is no doubt that when there is a single intravenous
immunization with the antigens mentioned above the initial period
of development of the immune process takes place under conditions
of a lowered level of mineralocorticoids in the blood.

Thus our own data and those reported in the literature confirm that the inductive phase of the immune process is accompanied by a stimulation of the glucocorticoid function of the HHAS; at the same time, particular influences may be exerted by physiologically active fractions of the corticosteroids. The same period of development of an immune reaction is characterized by a lowered concentration of mineralocorticoids, at least under conditions of intravenous introduction of the antigens we investigated. In the productive phase of the immune response, we did not observe regular changes in the glucocorticoid functions of the adrenal cortex, at least not following all the antigens used. The contradictory data of other authors, who observed definite and regularly appearing hormonal changes during this phase, may possibly be explained by the specific properties of the antigens they used.

To investigate mechanisms of hormonal changes in response to the injection of antigens, we immunized animals after excluding various regions of the hypothalamus. We know that the hypothalamus mediates reactions of the hypophyseal-adrenal system to many, or almost all, stimuli. Afferent pathways of influence of various stimuli on the HHAS can differ with the character of the stimulus, as is well known from the studies of the Stark laboratory (Budapest). The effects of most stimuli causing reaction of the HHAS are complex; these are brought about by humoral as well as neural pathways. In the final analysis, these and the other influences exhibit themselves as the hypothalamic neuroendocrine process of formation of the corticotropin-releasing factor (CRF) (Aleshin 1971; Lissák and Endröczi 1967; Shreiber 1963; Szentagothai et al. 1965).

However, as experiments have shown (Makara et al. 1969; Stark 1972), one can speak of stimuli of predominantly humoral or neural effect, depending on the afferent pathways involved in the reaction. Various structures of the hypothalamus apparently can participate to differing degrees in the reaction, depending on the nature of the stimulus.

We were interested, first of all, in to what extent the influence of antigenic stimuli on the HHAS is mediated by the posterior hypothalamic area. From the preceding chapter we know that this area is one of the structures of the hypothalamus most sensitive to antigens and capable of modulating the intensity of the immune process. By

comparing the influence of injury to the region of the posterior hypothalamus with that of injury to the anterior hypothalamic structure on the intensity of hormonal shifts caused by immunization, we hoped to establish the involvement of the posterior hypothalamic area in the hormonal response to the antigen. To form an opinion concerning the specificity of the changes observed for stimuli of antigenic origin, we used stimuli of different natures: immobilization (a stimulus of predominantly neuroreflex action); ethymisole (a preparation apparently having direct humoral effects on the hypothalamus) (Danilova et al. 1972; Ryzhenkov 1968); and horse serum (a stimulus of complex humoral nature starting a chain of reactions participating in the immune process and at the same time activating the HHAS (Shkhinek et al. 1973).

In most experimental animals, the foci of injury were in the posterior hypothalamic area, including to a small degree the boundary structures, whereas in control rabbits they were at the border of the medial and lateral preoptic regions.

Investigations showed (Shkhinek 1975a) that injuries in the region of the posterior hypothalamus lower the concentration of 11-OH-CS somewhat as contrasted with nonoperated rabbits (the changes are not statistically significant; $p > .05$). Injuries to the posterior hypothalamus, however, considerably change the reaction to all stimuli (figs. 30–32). On the 5th–7th days after injury to the posterior hypothalamic region, we observed a considerable rise in the intensity of the hormonal reactions to all stimuli, and the hormonal response to the administration of ethymisole remained strong in the following periods (10th, 15th, 25th days) in the absence of changes in nonoperated animals (fig. 32). Injury of the preoptic area of the hypothalamus had practically no influence on the intensity of the reactions in response to ethymisole, and immunization did not cause a significant lowering of the hormonal shift in response to horse serum (fig. 30). Thus it was established that the posterior hypothalamic area participates in the development of hormonal shifts in response to stimuli of antigenic and nonantigenic character. Since a rise in the intensity of reactions was noted regardless of the nature of the stimulus and the character of afferent pathways of its effect on the HHAS, one can assume that it is the central link of the reaction that is responsible for this effect, and the region of the hypothalamic

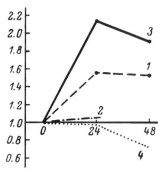

Fig. 30   Changes in the concentration of plasma 11-hydroxycorticosteroids
in response to administration of horse serum in rabbits immunized
after hypothalamic lesions: 1, intact immunized animals; 2, control
unimmunized animals; 3, animals immunized on the 5th–6th days
after lesions in the posterior hypothalamic area; 4, animals immunized on the 5th–6th days after lesions in the anterior preoptic area.
Abscissae, time (hours) after immunization, or corresponding time
in control group; ordinates, concentration of 11-hydroxycortico-
steroids with reference to the initial level, taken as 1.

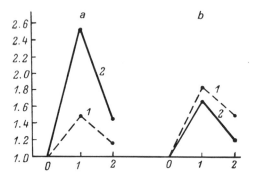

Fig. 31   Changes in the concentration of plasma 11-hydroxycorticosteroids
in rabbits in response to an hour-long immobilization before (1)
and after (2) hypothalamic lesions: a, animals with lesions in the
posterior hypothalamic area; b, animals with lesions in the anterior
preoptic area. Abscissae, time (hours) after the beginning of immobilization; ordinates, as in figure 30.

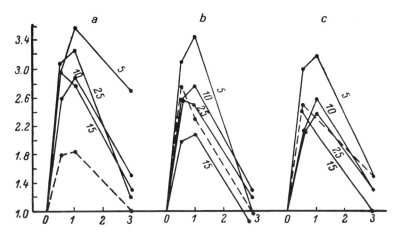

Fig. 32   Changes in the concentration of plasma 11-hydroxycorticosteroids in response to administration of ethymisole in rabbits before and at various times after hypothalamic lesions: *a,* animals with lesions in the posterior hypothalamic area; *b,* intact control animals; *c,* animals with lesions in the preoptic area. *Broken lines,* reaction before surgery; *solid lines,* reactions on various days (numbers) after surgery or on corresponding days in the control group. Abscissae, time (hours) after administration of ethymisole; ordinates, as in figure 30.

area has, possibly, a relation to the regulation of the release of CRF in response to stress stimuli.

However, in these experiments it was not possible to exclude the possibility of a neurotropic influence on the adrenal cortex from the injury of the hypothalamus, which could change the sensitivity of the endocrine gland itself to the endogenous ACTH. Further investigation showed no changes in the reaction of the adrenal cortex to exogenous corticotropin in a dosage of 3 units/kg in animals with injury to the posterior hypothalamic area. This confirmed the assumption concerning the major role of central mechanisms in disturbances of hormonal shifts after injury to the posterior hypothalamic area.

Taking into account the morphological data on connections of the posterior hypothalamic area with structures of the mesencephalon

and thalamus (Knigge and Skott 1970; Nauta 1960), the physiological data on the variability of hormonal responses elicited by electrical stimulation of this region (Shkhinek et al. 1967), and the hetero-directivity of the changes in the level of corticosteroids and intensity of hormonal reactions after its injury in our experiments, we can assume that the region of the posterior hypothalamic area includes elements participating in stimulating as well as inhibitory influences. Apparently a macroinjury disturbs the normal balance of these influences, and that is in the final analysis expressed in inappropriately intensified reactions of hormone release in response to various stimuli, including antigens, against a background of normal or even somewhat lowered levels of hormones in the resting state.

To understand the physiological role of hormonal changes observed in the development of immune reactions, it is important to investigate the correlations between the intensity of these hormonal shifts and the intensity of the immune response. However, up to now such an analysis has not been conducted. We attempted to investigate the interrelations of hormonal shifts accompanying the development of a hormonal immune response with the indexes of the intensity of antibody production. For this purpose we used three methods. First we made a comparative analysis of hormonal changes in the inductive phase in normal immunized animals with varying intensities of antibody production. Since the magnitude of the humoral immune response to the same antigen varied considerably in the individual rabbits in control groups, it was possible to compare the hormonal shifts in animals with relatively high and low antibody production. On the other hand, we compared the hormonal changes in animals with artificially suppressed and normal immune responses. For the depression of immune reactivity we used two models. The first model was stereotaxic electrolytic injury of the posterior hypothalamic area (during immunization of such animals, as was described in preceding chapters, one usually finds a certain percentage of animals with considerably lowered responses). The second model consisted of competing antigens resulting from administration of two types of heterologous erythrocytes (Taussig 1973). A third experimental approach was to compare the intensity of immune reactions in animals with a definitely changed hormonal reaction to the antigen with the intensity observed in normal immu-

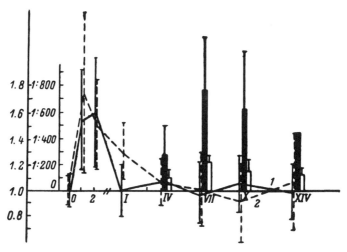

Fig. 33   Changes in the concentration of plasma 11-hydroxycorticosteroids in response to Vi-antigen of typhoid bacillus in control rabbits with different intensities of immune response: 1, 11-hydroxycorticosteroids in animals with high antibody titers (*solid bars*); 2, 11-hydroxycorticosteroids in animals with low antibody titers (*open bars.*) Abscissae, as in figure 27; ordinates on the left, concentration of 11-hydroxycorticosteroids with reference to the initial level, taken as 1; ordinates on the right, titers of hemagglutinins in diluted serum.

nized animals. To suppress the hormonal shift in response to the antigen, we administered a single dose of 4 mg/kg dexamethasone 3.5 hours after immunization. It is known that dexamethasone blocks the function of ACTH at the level of hypothalamus-hypophysis (Aleshin 1971; Lissak and Endröczi 1967).

An investigation of hormonal changes accompanying the development of immune reactions in control animals with different intensities of immune response was conducted in rabbits immunized with horse serum and Vi-antigen. We noted no real differences in hormonal shifts between rabbits with different intensities of antibody production (fig. 33), although the differences in the titers of antibodies were statistically significant (Shkhinek 1975b; Shkhinek et al. 1973).

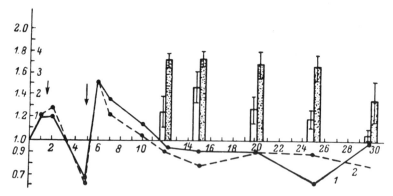

Fig. 34   Dynamics of concentration of 11-hydroxycorticosteroids in rabbits with different intensities of immune responses to horse serum, immunized after lesions in the posterior hypothalamic area. *First arrow,* surgery; *second arrow,* immunization. Abscissae, time (days) after surgery; ordinates, titers of complement-binding antibodies (arbitrary units). Other designations as in figure 33.

Of definite interest is the comparison of the indicators of the binding capability of transcortin in animals with different magnitudes of humoral immune reactions; these experiments were conducted on rabbits immunized with Vi-antigen. The indicators of the binding capability of transcortin were analyzed in three groups of animals with different antibody titers. According to these data, our impression is that in rabbits with the highest antibody titers, the indicators of the binding capability of transcortin are lowest; however, the differences were not statistically significant.

In experiments with suppression of the immune response by injuring the posterior hypothalamic area, we compared the changes in the concentrations of 11-OH-CS in blood plasma in operated rabbits with marked immunodepression and without the depressive effect. In spite of the definite differences in the dynamics of hormonal shifts between the operated and nonoperated animals, we did not detect reliable differences between the operated rabbits with depressed and normal antibody production (fig. 34). In both types of animals we saw an intensification of the hormonal response to horse serum during the inductive phase and an absence of a secondary rise

in the level of hormones on the 14th–20th days (characteristic for the control animals), after which the hormonal indicators returned to normal. Processing the data by the dispersion method did not make it possible to show reliable differences between the groups compared (Shkhinek et al. 1973). These data do not permit us to conclude that the changes in 11-OH-CS in the blood are the deciding factor in the inhibitory influences of injury to the posterior hypothalamus on the processes of antibody formation in rabbits.

Yet some authors investigating the role of hormones in the suppression of the humoral immune response caused by injury to the structures of the hypothalamic region expressed the assumption that in this phenomenon changes in the glucocorticoid function of the adrenal cortex may play a definite role (Filipp 1973; Filipp and Mess 1969a,b). It was established that, though hypophysectomy and adrenalectomy do not in themselves cause changes in antibody titers in rats, removing the glands does weaken the inhibitory effect of destruction of the anterior hypothalamic area on the humoral immune response (Tyrey and Nalbandov 1972). The authors assume that the effect on immunoproduction of destruction of hypothalamic structures results from increase in adrenocortical function. Since we found no essential differences in the level of hormones in operated animals with depressed and normal immune responses, we assume that hormonal changes observed as a response to an antigen in animals with injury of the region of the posterior hypothalamus area may facilitate the actions of other factors that participate in inhibiting antibody production but that in themselves are not sufficient to inhibit the immune process.

In another series of experiments on mice (Karasik and Shkhinek, unpublished data), the inhibition of the immune reaction was achieved through successive administration of two types of heterologous erythrocytes. Rat erythrocytes in a dosage of 2×10^7 per animal were administered on the 3d day after immunization with sheep erythrocytes in a dosage of 2×10^9. The immune response to the rat erythrocytes, evaluated by the reaction of agglutination in serum on the 6th day after immunization, was five times lower under these conditions compared with the reaction to rat erythrocytes alone. However, the content of 11-OH-CS in blood plasma, determined 2, 4, and 24 hours and 6 days after immunization, did not dif-

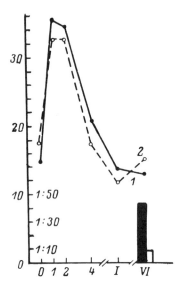

Fig. 35   Dynamics of concentration of plasma 11-hydroxycorticosteroids in
mice immunized with rat erythrocytes without preliminary administration (1) and on the 3d day after preliminary administration (2)
of sheep erythrocytes. *Solid bar,* antibody titers in group 1; *open
bar,* antibody titers in group 2. Abscissae, as in figure 28; ordinates
on the left, concentration of 11-hydroxycorticosteroids (μg/100
ml); ordinates on the right, hemagglutinin titers in diluted serum.

fer significantly in the groups of animals compared (fig. 35). Thus,
in this case also no direct correlation was detected between the intensity of the immune response and the magnitude of endogenous hormonal shifts accompanying the development of a hormonal immune
response (fig. 35).

In the series of experiments with dexamethasone blockage of the
HHAS, we achieved complete suppression of hormonal reaction to
the administration of Vi-antigen (fig. 36). However, the absence of a
rise in the 11-OH-CS concentration in response to the antigen did
not significantly influence the intensity of antibody production: the
differences in antibody titers were not statistically significant (fig.
36). A small tendency toward a decrease in the titers in the experimental group is probably due to the effect of dexamethasone itself
as a preparation possessing glucocorticoid properties.

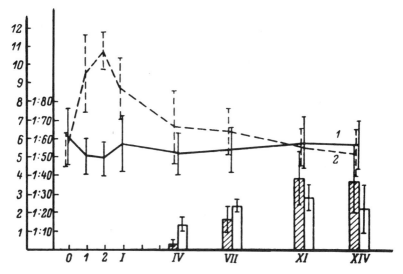

Fig. 36   Changes in the concentration of plasma 11-hydroxycorticosteroids
                 and in antibody titers in rabbits immunized after preliminary single
                 administration of dexamethasone (1) and without it (2). *Open bars,*
                 antibody titers in group 1; *striped bars,* antibody titers in group 2.
                 Other designations as in figure 28.

Thus, in this experimental model we established no clear correlation between the intensity of an increase in 11-OH-CS in response to the antigen in the inductive period and the magnitude of antibody production (fig. 36).

In examining the changes in the function of the HHAS in the formation of the primary immune response, we are concerned with the most elementary interrelations of nonspecific and specific factors of defense. These interrelations become considerably more complex with sensitization of the organism. Hypersensitive states (anaphylaxis as well as local and general allergic phenomena) are characterized by an exceedingly diverse and complex picture of neurohumoral and immune mechanisms, making it very difficult to analyze the origin of hormonal changes, particularly their role in the development of immune processes. Since the question has not been studied systematically, we cite here only some data on diverse forms of

manifestations of hypersensitivity. Long ago it was observed that adrenalectomy aggravates the course of allergic processes. In adrenalectomized animals, anaphylactic shock and other manifestations of hypersensitivity develop faster (Rose 1959). Some authors observed a concomitant rise in antibody production (Dews and Code 1953; Rose 1959), but as we pointed out above, the data on the influence of adrenalectomy on immune reactions are very contradictory.

In studies of the role of the CNS and hormones of the HHAS in anaphylaxis, it was established that there was a decrease in the inhibitory effects of injury to certain zones of the hypothalamus on the course of anaphylactic shock in adrenalectomized guinea pigs (Filipp and Mess 1969a). The conclusion is drawn that the hyperfunction of the adrenals is one of the major causes of suppression of the shock reaction in animals with destroyed hypothalamus. Yet, according to some data, hypophysectomy has no influence either on antibody production or on manifestation of anaphylaxis in operated animals, and injuries to the hypothalamus per se have no influence on these processes (Thatcher et al. 1948). A number of experiments established that the process of sensitization can be accompanied by a stimulation of the glucocorticoid functions of the adrenal cortex. During sensitization with horse serum and the development of anaphylaxis in dogs, the content of 17-hydroxycorticosteroid in blood plasma increased markedly following administration of a deciding dose of antigen (Yeremina et al. 1970).

An increase in the level of glucocorticoids in blood plasma of dogs has been observed in the process of sensitization with typhoid endotoxin and the development of a generalized Shwartzman phenomenon (Denisenko 1970) as well as in experimental allergic encephalitis in these animals (Khoruzhaya 1967). An increase in urinary 17-hydroxycorticosteroids was found during the development of the Arthus phenomenon in guinea pigs (Al'pern 1964). The initial period of sensitization with a weak pathogenic culture of streptococci during the production of experimental rheumatoid polyarthritis in rabbits in experiments by Astrauskas (Astrauskas 1968; Astrauskas and Leonavichene 1975; Astrauskas et al. 1963) also was accompanied by a rise in the glucocorticoid function of the adrenal cortex. However, a prolonged sensitization finally led to a lowering of the

level of hormones, although the function of the gland was not exhausted as would be expected if we see the development of this pathological state as a disturbance of adaptation.

Allergic processes are accompanied not only by changes in the content of glucocorticoids in blood plasma, but also by significant disturbances of their metabolism in tissues (Pytskaya 1970; Pytskiy 1969; Khoruzhaya and Vilkov 1970). It has been established that in sensitized animals bacterial and serum antigens depress the metabolism of cortisol in the liver (Pytskaya 1970). Pytskiy et al. (1972) consider that the functional and metabolic disturbances observed in allergic processes point to a glucocorticoid insufficiency that does not always become apparent by direct measurement of the level of hormones in blood plasma. Sources of such insufficiency can, in the authors' opinion, be a suppression of secretion of adrenal glucocorticoids in connection with a direct effect of allergens, the increase of binding capability of transcortin, lowering of the activity of corticoids in the tissues, and suppression of transformation of cortisol into cortisone in the liver as well as changes in the intensity of metabolism in the liver. Probably the diversity of models of hypersensitivity in which the hormonal shifts were studied in itself excludes identical results. Apparently a more systematic parallel study of hormonal, humoral, and immune indicators involved in definite forms of hypersensitivity can delineate the role of hormones in the genesis and development of these phenomena.

Summarizing the data on the interaction of endogenous hormones of the HHAS and immune processes in the organism, we should emphasize the following characteristic features of this interaction. Endogenous ACTH and adrenocortical hormones take part in the organism's reactions to foreign proteins: the regular changes in the concentrations of glucocorticoid hormones in the plasma in response to the administration of bacterial and nonbacterial antigens point to this. These changes are most clearly expressed during the inductive phase of the immune process, especially in the first hours after immunization, when we see not only a rise in the level of total glucocorticoids, but also an increase in the concentrations of physiologically active fractions of hormones, suggested by the decrease in binding capacity of plasma transcortin during this period. Following administration of some antigens, changes in the level of

glucocorticoids can be observed in the productive phase of an immune reaction.

The hormonal shifts caused by antigens are achieved with the participation of central nervous mechanisms. One of the structures involved in this reaction is the posterior hypothalamus, as is confirmed by the marked changes of hormonal reactions in animals immunized after injury to this area.

Analysis of the mechanisms of hormonal reactions in response to different types of stimuli has shown that the participation of the posterior hypothalamus in the development of hormonal reactions not only is specific for antigenic stimuli, but also occurs during hormonal changes in response to stimuli of different types, independent of the afferent pathways of their action on the hypothalamus. Since antigens apparently do not penetrate the blood-brain barrier, one may hypothesize that they may act on the CNS reflexively or through some kind of humoral mediator causing changes in the functional state of certain central nervous structures, including the posterior hypothalamus. In the final analysis, the nervous impulses are transformed into a neurohumoral process of CRF release, stimulating the production of ACTH, which leads to a rise in synthesis and release of glucocorticoids by cells of the adrenal cortex. This hormonal shift takes place almost at once after the antigen enters the organism; however, it is not clear to what extent the presence of antigen is necessary for the further development of the reaction, since the relation between the duration and intensity of the hormonal changes and the length of time the antigen has been in the organism has not been investigated.

The physiological role of hormonal shifts during the inductive phase is as yet not sufficiently clear. As was established in the experiments described above, their intensity did not correlate with the magnitude of the humoral immune response either in control animals with varying intensities of immune reactions or in animals with artificially suppressed immune responses. These data make it possible to conclude that changes in the functional activity of the HHAS do not in themselves regulate the magnitude of humoral immune reactions. They can, apparently, play a secondary role in the activities of other factors that are more definitely and directly connected with immune processes. It is possible, as Belovolova (1973) and Polyak et

al. (1974) assume, that these hormonal changes, together with other humoral factors, participate in the preparation of the immune system and the synthesis of antibodies.

But what is the specific role of ACTH or the glucocorticoids in this process? As was shown above, variations in the level of hormones in response to the administration of antigens were comparatively small: they amounted, on the average, to 45–150% of control levels. As we mentioned in evaluating the influence of exogenous hormones, it is difficult to imagine that such shifts can cause a depressive effect on the humoral response of the immune system as a whole. For such an effect large doses of steroids are needed, tens and hundreds of times exceeding the physiological level.

Experiments with various types of stress showed that producing a depressive effect of endogenous steroids on a humoral response of the system takes an intensive and prolonged influence. Consequently it is difficult to expect that the endogenous hormonal shifts caused by antigens can inhibit the work of the whole system. This would apparently contradict the physiological sense of the reaction to an antigen, since its final result is to stimulate antibody synthesis. It would be more natural to assume that comparatively small hormonal shifts, observed in the inductive phase, together with other neural and humoral factors, facilitate the activation of cells of the immunocompetent system. There are some bases for such an assumption.

As we stated above, according to data obtained in vitro, the humoral immune response in some models cannot be achieved in the absence of glucocorticoids, and physiological concentrations of these hormones in the culture medium cause not a depression but a stimulation of antibody formation. Of course, in the organism it may be much more complex. However, it is difficult to conceive that in the absence of glucocorticoids the immune response could occur normally. Unfortunately, data obtained from adrenalectomized animals, in view of their contradictions, cannot confirm this assumption accurately enough. Apparently only a selective pharmacologic exclusion of glucocorticoid function in the organism could elucidate its role in the formation of immune reactions (one must, of course, take into account the instances where there is no directly depressing effect of the preparation itself on the immune reactions).

Considering various pathways of the effect of glucocorticoids on immunocompetent tissues in the organism, it is appropriate to remember the possibility of the permissive effect of physiological concentrations of these hormones established in relation to general metabolic effects (Leytes 1964; Ingle 1954) as well as with respect to their influences on the synthesis of antibodies in lymphocyte tissue cultures (Ambrose 1970). We can assume that in the organism changes in the level of hormones in the inductive phase, though not in themselves influencing the level of antibody production, also have a permissive effect on other factors more directly connected with this process. Thus at present it is permissible only to conjecture hypothetically concerning the role of endogenous shifts in concentrations of glucocorticoids accompanying the development of immune reactions.

Note that in studying the changes in concentration of glucocorticoids in various phases of the immune process we exclude them artificially from the general neurohumoral shift that also includes the changes in the content of biogenic amines (Belovolova 1973; Devoyno 1975; Kozlov 1968; Polyak et al. 1974; Frolov, 1974) and other hormones. Indeed, in response to many stressors, as we already pointed out, one observes the release not only of corticosteroids but also of mineralocorticoids, somatropin, thyrotropin, and sex hormones. Probably the antigens as stressors are no exception, so that the hormones above also react to the entry of foreign protein into the organism. In such a manner a whole complex of neurohumoral factors with complex interrelations between its components influences the immune system in the inductive phase. Therefore, to evaluate the physiological role of each of the humoral or hormonal agents participating in the reaction to the antigen, we must investigate the interrelations between them.

As we noted, some authors (Belovolova 1973; Polyak et al. 1974) found regular changes in the concentration of glucocorticoids together with changes in the concentration of catecholamines and histamine, not only in the inductive phase but also in the productive phase of immune response. They thus assume that the phase changes of the neurohumoral factors are determined, first of all, by the stages of the process of immunogenesis itself. Administering antigens

causes a state of stress manifesting itself in a rise in the activity of the sympathoadrenal and adrenopituitary systems and of histaminergic structures, all of whose hormones and mediators participate actively in the preparation of morphofunctional changes in the system of immunogenesis (i.e., in the cells of immunocompetent tissues).

Antibody synthesis functions of the immunocompetent system and the process of antibody development, in the opinion of these authors, in their turn activate the factors of neurohumoral regulation by the central control apparatus. We fully share their point of view concerning the possible role of neurohumoral changes during the inductive phase of preparing the immune system for its specific activity; however, we cannot agree with their interpretation of the neurohumoral changes in the productive phase, at least not with respect to ACTH and glucocorticoids. Since not every antigen changes the function of the HHAS in the productive phase, it is not justifiable to draw conclusions concerning the stimulating influence of the formation of an antibody synthetic function and of the process of antibody formation on factors of neurohumoral regulation in general. It is possible that this statement is correct only for processes caused by certain antigens and in regard only to certain types of humoral shifts, not for all immune processes caused by any particular antigen.

In studying the influence of endogenous corticosteroids on immune processes, we must distinguish between the role of hormonal changes in the development of an immune reaction due to the antigen itself and the influence of changes in the endogenous endocrine balance caused by other stimuli. If in the first case we do not find correlations between the magnitude of the endocrine increase (usually not very marked) and the intensity of the humoral response of the immune system, and if we assume that the hormonal shifts here play some kind of supporting role for the actions of the other factors that stimulate immune reactions, then in the second case of sufficiently intensive and prolonged influence, it is probable that the hormones per se depress the immune response. Experiments with some types of stress demonstrate this.

Evidently, as with the effect of exogenous hormones, the character of the influence of the endogenous hormonal shift depends on the intensity of this shift, the specific properties and dosage of the

administered antigen, and, as the data cited above showed, on the time the disturbances of hormonal balance appear relative to immunization. As in the experiments with the use of exogenous hormones, it has been established that the observed changes of concentration of glucocorticoids during stress cause a more marked depression of the humoral immune response and the functions of individual lymphoid cells if they act several hours before immunization. This is confirmed by data obtained from administration of exogenous hormones: the first stages of the immune process, which apparently are connected with the activity of antigen-sensitive elements, are most sensitive to variations in the level of hormones.

Note that, as in the experiments with exogenous hormones, there is a definite dissociation between the depressive influence of endogenous hormones on the lymphocytes and their influence on the humoral immune response of the whole system. Although some authors observed a depressing effect on the immune activity of certain populations of lymphoid cells from a single application of stressors, a depressive effect on the *humoral* immune response was very difficult to obtain even from a repeated application of different types of stressors, particularly with certain types of stressors. It appears that not all populations of immunocompetent cells respond identically to changes in endogenous hormones; this may determine the differences between humoral immune responses of the whole system and changes in the functions of cells of certain parts of this system.

Of course stressors by their very nature exert complex effects. Therefore the data obtained should not be considered as relating only to changes in the concentration of corticosteroids. The findings on how different types of stressors influence immune processes evidently can demonstrate the effect of corticosteroids only when the total effects of various other factors are taken into account.

Sex Hormones and the Immune Response

The influence of sex steroids and also the role of endogenous sex hormones on immune reactions have received very little study.

Administering exogenous sex hormones in large enough doses inhibits humoral and cellular immune responses. This is shown in regard to chorionic gonadotropins (Speranskiy 1972; Speranskiy and

Muslyumova 1974; Beling and Weksler 1974; Han 1974a,b; Jones and Kayc 1973), estrogens (Shemerovskaya 1974; Slyivic et al. 1975), and testosterone (Katani et al. 1974). Yurina et al. (1975) noted complex influences of estrogens on cellular systems of the blood and connective tissue participating in the immune response: sinestrol led to the development of lymphopenia and eosinopenia in blood and bone marrow; however, the content of plasma cells in the lymph nodes and bone marow was markedly increased. This preparation had the same effect on immunized animals.

Chorionic gonadotropins can inhibit the reaction of lymphocyte blast transformation caused by phytohemagglutinin or other mitogenic stimuli (Han 1974a,b, 1975). The same effect was observed for estrogens: prolactin (Karmali et al. 1974) and diethylstilbestrol (Ablin et al. 1974a,b). The inhibiting effect of chorionic gonadotropins and estradiol on the reaction of blast transformation can be related to a lowered inclusion of labeled amino acids in desoxyribonucleic acid, which suggests a decrease in its synthesis (Ablin et al. 1974b; Han 1974b). The inhibiting effect of chorionic gonadotropins on the development of the blastogenic reaction in response to mitogenic stimuli or antigens depends on the dosage of the hormone: it appears only in response to rather high doses (Han 1974a,b).

Sex steroids inhibit the development of thymus and peripheral lymphatic tissues in mice and rats (Cherry et al. 1967; Reilly et al. 1967; Sherman et al. 1964; Thompson et al. 1967; Warner and Burnet 1961). The cells of the bursa of Fabricius in chick embryos apparently possess a selective capacity for accumulating labeled testosterone that leads to their selective elimination (Glick and Schwarz 1975). Kostinskiy (1975) showed that androgens administered to young rats (1–40 days old) cause a dose-dependent inhibition of the humoral immune response to sheep erythrocytes.

Castration intensifies the humoral immune response in adult male mice and also increases the weights of the thymus and lymph nodes. Castration in conjunction with thymectomy does not lead to an increase in the size of the lymph nodes. The absolute number of lymphocytes increases under the influence of castration (Castro 1973, 1974). Castro thinks that castration, by lowering the level of androgens, increases the immune response at the expense of growth in the number of T-cells.

There is a complex functional interconnection in the activities of the thymus and sex glands in mice. Gonadectomy decreased hypoplasia of the lymphatic structures of the spleen and lymph nodes in neonatal thymectomized mice, but it did not influence the deficit in humoral immune responses caused by thymectomy (Pierpaoli and Sorkin 1968b).

The cited investigations of the influence of sex steroids on immune reactions do not make it possible to come to definite conclusions concerning either the dependence of these hormones on dosages and time of administration relative to immunization or the role of exogenous or endogenous hormones on immune processes.

Somatotropin, Thyrotropin, Hormones of the Thyroid Gland, and the Immune Response

Although at present there are comparatively few investigations devoted to the influence of somatotropin, thyrotropin, and hormones of the thyroid gland, their results offer rather definite conclusions in regard to the character of the effect of these hormones on the immune capabilities of the organism, especially the interconnections between these endocrine factors and the immune system during early ontogenesis.

The influence of exogenous somatotropin, thyrotropin, and the hormones of the thyroid gland has been established in several experiments. Administering somatotropin to the organism can stimulate humoral as well as cellular immune reactions. However, this effect is manifested in adult animals only under certain experimental conditions. Somatotropin causes a reactivation of the plasmocyte reaction and the formation of agglutinins in lymph nodes in previously immunized rats (Zdrodovskiy 1962, 1971; Zdrodovskiy and Gurvich 1972; Zdrodovskiy et al. 1973). In these experiments the hormone was administered at the end of the productive phase. Shemerovskaya (1974) observed an intensification of the humoral immune response and reactions of hypersensitivity of the slow type following the administration of somatotropin during different stages of the development of the immune process; however, the stimulating influence of somatotropin on cellular and humoral immune processes depended on the dose of the antigen. Somatotropin considerably stimulated the humoral immune response to sheep erythrocytes

in guinea pigs only if small threshold doses of the antigen were used. The same regularity was observed in the influence of somatotropin on the development of hypersensitivity of the slow type to tuberculosis mycobacteria. The author suggests that these differences may be connected with the stimulating effect of optimal doses of antigens on the production of endogenous somatotropin, which does not permit the influence of the exogenous hormone to appear. Somatotropin increases the production of antibodies to virus antigens (Izotov and Lazarev 1963), and it can influence the processes of immune memory while the period of sensitization is most sensitive to the hormone and the period of memory storage is intact to the effect of the hormone (Shemerovskaya and Kovaleva 1975).

Hayashida and Li (1957), however, did not observe marked effects of somatotropin on antibody formation in normal adult rats, although they observed an opposite effect in regard to the immunodepressive actions of ACTH. Holne et al. (1954) detected hyperplasia of the spleen and thymus following administration of somatotropin to rats for 7 days before immunization; however, the titers of hemolytic antibodies fell. Administering a combination of somatotropin and hydrocortisone in doses ensuring normal growth led to normal levels of antibody production. These authors suggest that for an optimal production of antibodies in the organism a good equilibrium in the level of glucocorticoids and somatotropin is essential.

The influence of somatotropin on the immune response is apparently connected, first of all, with the capability of this hormone to intensify proliferative processes in thymus, spleen, and lymph nodes (Zdrodovskiy 1962, 1971; Zdrodovskiy and Gurvich 1972; Lundin 1958; Schellin et al. 1954). The changes in the cells of the lymphoid system caused by somatotropin have a persistent character; the stimulating humoral and cellular immune response effects of the hormone are retained even after transfer of lymphoid cells to recipients (Shemerovskaya 1974). As was shown in other experiments involving transfer, somatotropin affects the transformation of precursor cells into T-cells but has no influence on differentiated T-cells.

The effects of growth hormone on immune processes at the molecular level are apparently related primarily to its stimulating influence on protein synthesis (Zdrodovskiy 1962, 1971; Zdrodovskiy

and Gurvich 1972; Glick et al. 1965). Indeed, somatotropin has a marked anabolic effect and substantially influences other types of metabolism (Balabolkin 1971). In the mechanisms of interaction of somatotropin with cells of the lymphoid system, the kinetic processes of binding the hormone with protein apparently play an important role. It has been shown that lymphocytes have specific receptors for growth hormone (Lesniak et al. 1973). Some authors (Hanjan and Talwar 1975) attach great significance to the interaction of growth hormone with cyclic adenomonophosphate in its influence on cellular metabolism, including that of lymphoid cells (Maor et al. 1974). There are some direct data on the stimulating influence of endogenous somatotropin on immune processes in the adult organism. We should mention, first of all, the depressive effect of antisomatotropic serum on the development of the immune reaction. Such an effect was obtained in rats immunized with sheep erythrocytes. Administering antisomatotropic horse serum markedly suppressed the number of antibody-forming cells in the spleen (Zdrodovskiy 1971; Zdrodovskiy and Gurvich 1972). The depressing influence of antisomatotropic serum on the synthesis of antibodies and the involution of lymphoid tissue in adult and young mice has been established (Pierpaoli and Sorkin 1968c, 1969a; Sorkin and Pierpaoli 1970).

On the basis of these data, we can conclude that somatotropin is essential in regulating immune reactions in the adult organism and as a stimulator of processes of protein synthesis in general and synthesis of immunoglobulins in particular (Zdrodovskiy 1971; Zdrodovskiy and Gurvich 1972).

Studies of the influence of thyrotropin and hormones of the thyroid gland on immune reactions have shown that the hormones of this system also are related to the formation of reactions of specific defense. Exogenous thyroidin and thyroxin apparently stimulate the lymphoid system in adult animals. Adamov and Nikolayev (1968) reported an intensification of antibody production in rabbits under the influence of thyroidin. Thyroxin significantly raised the humoral response to sheep erythrocytes in normal rats (Fabris and Corda 1973). Thyroxin had no significant influence on antibody production in response to smallpox vaccine in rabbits, but it intensified the phagocytic activity of the reticuloendothelial system in experiments

by Mikaelyan et al. (1972a,b). An intensification of phagocytic activity following administration of hormones of the thyroid gland was found by Kebadze (1957). Exogenous thyroxin caused hypertrophy of central and peripheral lymphoid organs and an increase in the release of small lymphocytes from the thymus (Ernstrom and Larson 1966).

Endogenous hormones of the thyroid gland act on the lymphoid system in a similar manner. Hyperthyroid patients show proliferation of lymphoid tissues as well as an increase in the number of lymphocytes in peripheral blood (Ultman et al. 1963). Thyroidectomy in adult rats decreases the absolute and relative weights of thymus, lymph nodes, and spleen, though this effect is not large. Thyroidectomy decreases the number of lymphocytes in peripheral blood and the number of patch-forming cells in the spleen and lowers the humoral immune response to sheep erythrocytes. The proliferative capacities of the spleen cells in response to phytohemagglutinin are also lowered by thyroidectomy. Administering thyroxin fully restores the deficiencies caused by thyroidectomy (Fabris 1973). Thyroidectomy inhibits antibody formation and development of a plasmocytic reaction in response to immunization with various antigens (Ass-Babich 1966; Mikaelyan et al. 1972a,b; Sakanyan et al. 1972a,b,c).

The inhibiting effect of hormone insufficiency of the thyroid gland on immune reactions may depend on the duration and magnitude of the hormone deficit. Chaplinskiy (1973) noticed that a brief administration of methylthiouracil, a substance that depresses the excretion of thyroxin, leads first not to an inhibition but a stimulation of phagocytic activity of leukocytes, and only after prolonged administration is there a depressive effect on these reactions and on antibody synthesis.

The data above indicate a possible role of somatotropin, thyrotropin, and hormones of the thyroid gland in the achievement of immune reactions in adult animals. However, certain factors are particularly important for the development of immune capabilities during the period of postnatal ontogenesis. Experiments on animals with congenital immunodeficient states caused by underdeveloped hypophyses have made a great contribution to solving this problem.

In hypohypophyseal dwarf mice, a marked hypotrophy of the thymus and peripheral lymphoid tissue was observed, which led to

decreased immune reactivity (Baroni 1967; Baroni et al. 1967; Du-gueskoy et al. 1970; Fabris et al. 1970; Pierpaoli et al. 1969; Pierpaoli and Sorkin 1968a). The production of somatotropin and thyroxin in such animals was markedly lowered (Pierpaoli et al. 1969). Administering somatotropin and thyrotropin restored immune capability in these animals (Fabris et al. 1970; Pierpaoli et al. 1969) but did not normalize them in the absence of the thymus (Fabris et al. 1970). Lowering the level of somatotropin and thyrotropin with the appropriate antisera led to similar changes in the structure of the thymus and peripheral lymphoid tissues and in young mice caused an inhibition of antibody production similar to that observed in hypohypophyseal dwarfs (Us 1973; Pierpaoli and Sorkin 1968c, 1969a,b). Somatotropin and thyrotropin corrected the defects caused by antisera; even somatotropin alone can normalize the disturbed immune capabilities (Pierpaoli et al. 1969). Somatotropin restored functions of the lymphoid tissues disturbed by the administration of antithyrotropic serum (Pierpaoli et al. 1969).

Thus, on the one hand, it has been convincingly shown that the organism's development of lymphoid tissue and its immune capabilities are absolutely dependent on hypophyseal and thyroid hormones. At the same time, it was also established that the thymus can influence the development of the hypophysis. Neonatal thymectomy caused changes in the acidophilic cells of the hypophysis, which produce somatotropin (Pierpaoli and Sorkin 1967; 1969a); and somatotropin is a factor regulating the maturation and functional activity of thymus cells. Consequently there is a close interconnection between the functions of the hypophysis and the thymus. Sorkin and Pierpaoli (1970) suggest that the interrelations between the thymus and hypophysis play a most important role in the maturation of immune capabilities of the lymphoid system (fig. 37). These hormones, in their opinion, regulate the distribution of cells of the thymus and the high level of mitosis in this organ during the growth period of the organism before and after sexual maturity.

Conclusion

Investigations of the influence of endocrine factors on immune processes were limited until recently to the study of the effects of exogenous hormones. In regard to some of them (primarily hormones

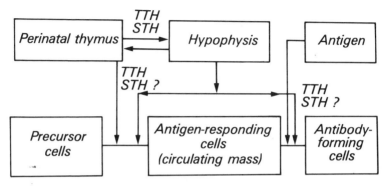

Fig. 37   Schema of neuroendocrine and immune system interactions, ac-
                  cording to Sorkin and Pierpaoli (1970). STH, somatotropic hor-
                  mone; TTH, thyrotropic hormone.

of the HHAS), data were obtained making it possible to evaluate the
influence of exogenous hormones on the immune system as a whole
and also on possible mechanisms of their effects at cellular and subcellular levels. These investigations made an important contribution
to the concept of possible hormonal intervention in the regulation of
immune processes. However, up to the present practically only one
type of hormonal intervention has been used in medical practice,
namely, large doses of glucocorticoids to suppress immune reactivity
and various manifestations of hypersensitivity. It is this aspect of the
effect of glucocorticoids that has been most studied. However, effects of pharmacologic doses, in vivo as well as in vitro, do not give
an exact concept of how endocrine and immune processes interrelate
under physiological conditions of formation of immune reactivity.
At the same time, a knowledge of the mechanisms of this interaction
is necessary if we are to develop more rational methods of intervention in the course of specific protective reactions.

At present we can consider it established that the entry of antigen
into the organism causes, aside from its direct influence on the cells
of the immunocompetent system, a multiple complex of neurohumoral shifts. Important components of this complex are neuromediator and endocrine reactions. The role of neuromediators of sympathetic and parasympathetic origin and other biogenic amines in

the development of immune reactivity has been convincingly demonstrated in some recent investigations. It has been established that specific immune reactions can be stimulated by a predominance of sympathetic factors, whereas inhibition involves parasympathetic influences. Activating serotonergic structures inhibits the production of humoral antibodies and cellular immune reactions.

One of the most important links in neurohumoral reactions to antigens is represented by neuroendocrine shifts. These in turn are complex and, apparently, include a change of functions in a number of endocrine organs. Study of hormonal functions in the dynamics of the development of the immune process and their specific role in the regulation of this process began rather recently. Therefore it is difficult to evaluate the significance of changes in the general hormonal balance for the development of specific immune reactions. Only the degree of participation of certain components of the general endocrine shift in the development of these reactions can be analyzed.

One of the components of the neurohumoral complex associated with the development of immune processes is represented by changes in the function of the HHAS, which was demonstrated in particular in systematic stimulation of glucocorticoid functions of the adrenal cortex in response to antigens. This stimulation is most clearly observed during the inductive phase, during which there is an increase in physiologically active fractions of hormones. The hormonal shifts evoked during the inductive phase of the immune process are mediated in part by the nervous system, particularly the hypothalamic region. It is still not known by which pathways antigens act on the HHAS. Apparently, neuroreflex as well as humoral pathways are involved; the latter must be chiefly indirect, since it is known that most antigens do not penetrate the blood-brain barrier. Some antigens may be able to act directly on cells of the endocrine glands, especially when massive doses are administered.

As our investigations have shown, not all zones of the hypothalamus play an equal role in the reactions of the HHAS to antigens. The posterior hypothalamic area apparently has a connection with this process, in contrast to the anterior preoptic zone. However, the observed effect is not connected with specific properties of the antigen stimulus, since it also appears in response to different types of

stimuli. This supports the proposition about the mediating effects of antigens on the hypothalamus; however, the mediating mechanisms may be common to stimuli of antigenic and nonantigenic nature.

In the final analysis, neural and humoral influences on cells of the hypothalamus, according to current theories (Aleshin 1971; Eskin 1968; Lissak and Endröczi 1967; Shreiber 1963), are transformed on the basis of an increase in hypothalamic stimulation of the adrenal cortex in response to antigens, stimulating the synthesis of ACTH and consequently also glucocorticoids. However, the nonspecific character of the changes in the glucocorticoid fraction of the adrenal cortex in response to antigenic stimuli does not attest to the nonspecificity of the general hormonal shift in response to antigens. Since the spectra of hormonal changes in response to various stressors differ, as some recent studies have shown (Gisler et al. 1971), one can expect that further investigations will elucidate specific features of the humoral changes in response to antigens.

Most complex and at the same time most important is the question of what role is played by the changes in the concentration of glucocorticoids evoked by antigens in the development of humoral immune reactions. Since antigens cause comparatively small deviations in the content of hormones from the resting level, it is difficult to assume that they can inhibit the development of immune reorganization of lymphoid cells. In support of this statement are the facts that: (1) the inhibiting effects of corticosteroids are dose dependent, as has been shown in experiments with exogenous corticosteroids, and (2) it is rather difficult to inhibit humoral immune reactions in response to various stressors. It is easier to assume that the stimulation of glucocorticoid functions caused by antigens can, in combination with other neurohumoral factors, promote the functional reorganization of lymphoid cells for participation in the immune process. From experiments conducted in vitro, we know that the glucocorticoids in physiological concentrations not only do not inhibit the humoral response, but are essential for the normal process of antibody production in some immune models. It is possible that in the intact organism also, certain ranges of hormone concentrations can have not an inhibiting, but a stimulating effect on humoral immune reactions.

However, comparative analysis of the intensity of hormonal reactions in the inductive phase and the magnitude of the humoral immune response did not show direct correlations between these processes. In other words, the intensity of hormonal changes caused by the antigen in the inductive phase was not directly correlated with the magnitude of the immune response, either in the normal course of an immune reaction or when it was inhibited by various factors. This indicates that variations in the concentrations of hormones have no direct effect on the magnitude of antibody production caused by the antigen. We may assume that glucocorticoids can exert a permissive effect with respect to other factors that more directly influence the intensity of antibody production—for example, catecholamines. The possibility of permissive effects of corticosteroids has been established experimentally.

The inductive phase of the development of immune reactions is, on the one hand, most sensitive to the inhibiting effect of high doses of glucocorticoids; but on the other hand, physiological concentrations of these hormones are essential for the normal course of the immune process. This leads to the conclusion that cell elements reacting to antigen have a greater sensitivity to glucocorticoids than do antibody-producing cells. As we know, according to present concepts, stem hematopoietic elements, T- and B-lymphocytes, and macrophages participate in the immune process (Miller 1975; Unanue 1975). Dose-dependent effects of glucocorticoids have been observed in regard to all these elements. As was shown above, apparently the effect of hormones is manifested more strongly on T-lymphocytes than on the lymphocytes of bone-marrow origin. T-lymphocytes and macrophages are capable of restoring the immune response of cells in vitro that was disturbed by glucocorticoids (Lee et al. 1975). All these data attest that the initial stage of development of humoral immune responses, characterized by the interaction of macrophages and T- and B-lymphocytes, is particularly sensitive to hormonal links of the immune process.

It is possible that in the development of immune reactions in the intact organism as well these cells are the primary targets of the effects of physiological concentrations of hormones. In support of this proposition are the data indicating that stressors have their most

marked effects on immune reactivity of lymphoid cells and on humoral responses of the organism during the preinductive and inductive periods.

The intensity and duration of the hormonal shifts apparently play an important role in determining the nature of the effects of endogenous glucocorticoids on immune reactions. Only very large changes in the concentrations of hormones inhibit the development of immune processes. However, correlation of the degree of hormonal changes with intensity of immune reactions under these conditions has been insufficiently studied, particularly in regard to humoral immune reactions in the intact organism. Contradictory data on the influence of hormones on cellular and humoral immune reactions indicate that different subpopulations of lymphocytes vary in sensitivity to changes in the level of endogenous hormones, in a manner similar to their responses to exogenous hormones. Perhaps this explains the difficulty of inhibiting the humoral immune response in the intact organism, in contrast to the comparative ease of detecting changes in immune reactivity of individual cellular elements in certain zones of the lymphoid system under the influence of the same factors.

A point of controversy is the role of changes in the functions of the HHAS observed during the productive phase of the immune reaction. Some authors found systematic changes in the concentrations of glucocorticoids not only during the inductive phase, but also during the productive phase of the immune reaction. They developed the point of view that, together with other humoral shifts (changes in the concentrations of catecholamines and histamine), the corticosteroids exert a regulating influence on the course of immune processes during this phase. However, shifts in the glucocorticoid function of the adrenal cortex during immune reactions were not elicited by all antigens. Therefore, in our view it is premature to consider these changes as regulating the immune process in general.

Neuroendocrine reactions to antigens are, naturally, not limited to shifts in the concentrations of glucocorticoids. Very likely, in reaction to any strong stimulus, the system can also mobilize other endocrine functions. Shifts are possible in the concentrations of a great variety of hormones. However, at present we do not have direct data on the changes in the levels of various hormones in the dy-

namics of the development of immune processes. Therefore one can only speculate on how far these hormones participate in the development of immune reactions. It is important to note that, in the final analysis, the influence of hormonal shifts caused by antigens probably depends not on each of the components individually, but on their interactions and their balance.

Data on the influence of exogenous hormones give a basis for assuming that somatotropin, thyrotropin, thyroxin, sex steroids, and mineralocorticoids may participate in the neurohumoral regulation of immune processes. Exogenous mineralocorticoids in certain doses can stimulate immune reactions. Somatotropin is capable of stimulating immune responses in mature animals; this effect is particularly marked on an immune response of weak intensity, produced, for example, by threshold doses of an antigen. Excluding the effect of hormones of the thyroid gland in mature animals inhibits the immune response, which can be restored by administering thyroxin. A very important role is played by somatotropin, thyrotropin, and thyroxin in the maturation of the immune system during early ontogenesis. A deficit of these hormones in newborn or young, growing animals leads to acute hypoplasia in the thymus and in peripheral lymphoid tissues and lowers immune reactivity. This has been clearly demonstrated in animals with congenital insufficiency of the hypophysis as well as in animals receiving antisera to corresponding hormones. Note that a close interrelation exists between the developing thymus and hypophysis: underdevelopment of one organ leads to underdevelopment of the other. This testifies to the importance of the role of humoral factors of the thymus in the development of the hypophysis.

Taking into account current data on the regulation of somatotropin, thyrotropin, and gonadotropin, one can assume that if these hormones are involved in reactions of the organism to antigens, then this occurs in the same manner with hormones of the adrenal cortex (with the participation of central neural structures and particularly the hypothalamus).

The assumed and known interrelations between the hormonal and immune systems in the organism during the formation of immune reactivity, at the present stage of study, can be presented in the following manner. The entry of antigen into the organism stimulates

the hypothalamus, either reflexly or by the reflexive effect of some mediating humoral factors. This in turn leads to complex hormonal shifts that may include several components:

1. Release of ACTH by the hypophysis and of glucocorticoids by the adrenal cortex, which has been demonstrated experimentally.

2. Changes in the levels of mineralocorticoids (?). A possible influence of these hormones on immune reactions has been established in experiments with exogenous hormones.

3. Changes in the levels of somatotropin (?). Stimulating influences of this hormone on immune reactions are well demonstrated in the period of postnatal development, as well as in adult animals in experiments with exogenous hormones.

4. Changes in the release of thyrotropin and hormones of the thyroid gland (?). The role of these hormones in the formation of immune reactions has been established in the postnatal period of development, as well as in experiments on thyroidectomized adult animals.

5. Changes in the production of gonadotropins and corresponding sex hormones (?). A possible role of these hormones in the immune response has been shown following exogenous administration, as well as in some experiments on gonadectomized adult animals.

The influence of hormones is evidently directed primarily toward antigen-sensitive elements of the lymphoid system and the interrelations of cells during the first stages of development of an immune reaction. This can ensure optimal conditions for the interactions mentioned above and, consequently, for the subsequent proliferation of B-cells and the synthesis of antibodies by antibody-forming cells. However, the effect of hormones on subsequent stages of development of an immune response as well cannot be ruled out. This is shown by the fact that it is possible to change the immune response by administering exogenous hormones during the productive phase. Cells reacting to antigens can, by way of humoral products formed as a result of meeting an antigen, in their turn influence the hypothalamus. One may assume that the antibody-forming cells, via the products of their activity, complete the cycle by secondary actions on the hypothalamus; however, this requires experimental verification. The feedback between the perinatal thymus and hypophysis

(possibly achieved through interaction between hormones of the hypophysis and thymus) is well documented.

Probably only further careful study of the interrelations between endocrine functions and immune processes can give a better understanding of the role of hormones in forming immune reactivity in the organism and, consequently, lead to methods of rational therapeutic hormonal intervention in immune processes. Such investigations, from our point of view, can be conducted in the following basic directions.

First of all, it is necessary to study more fully the spectra of hormonal changes in the blood and various tissues accompanying the development of an immune response. Thus far, in this regard, only the glucocorticoid hormones of the adrenal cortex have been studied to any extent. Changes in the levels of somatotropin, thyrotropin, hormones of the thyroid gland, mineralocorticoids, and other hormones during different periods of development of a normal or experimentally changed immune response have not been investigated.

To elucidate the role of hormonal factors in the development of immune processes, it would be useful to study parameters of immune responses in experimental models with endogenous hypo- and hyperhormonal states. In this regard satisfactory studies have been conducted only with certain hormones of the hypophysis during early ontogenesis. Especially useful, from our point of view, would be investigations using pharmocologic agents to block the synthesis and release of hormones in corresponding glands or at the level of central regulating mechanisms. The possibilities of such methods of inhibiting endogenous functions have been well shown for hormones of the adrenal cortex (Komissarenko and Reznikov 1972) and for certain other hormones.

One of the interesting directions for further research at the cellular level appears to be the study of specific binding of hormones by cell receptors of the cells of immunocompetent tissues in the development of immune responses. Inasmuch as the binding of hormones by protein structures of cells has a direct relation to their influence on protein metabolism, we may expect correlations between immune reactivity of cells and processes of specific hormonal binding. Regarding research at the molecular level, of greatest interest would be the study of how endogenous hormones influence the metabolism

of cyclic nucleotides, which are, as we know, reactive to the effects of hormones as well an antigens.

Inasmuch as neurohumoral shifts accompanying the development of immune reactions in the organism include not only changes in the functional activity of the nervous system and hormonal balance, but also complex disturbances in the metabolism of biogenic amines, it is also necessary to investigate interactions between hormonal influences and the effects of biogenic amines on the immunocompetent systems at various levels. The latter aspect is especially important for clarifying mechanisms of hypersensitive states that are characterized by marked shifts in hormonal balance, as well as in the metabolism of biogenic amines.

These directions for research, of course, do not exhaust all possible variants of the investigation of the interrelations between the hormonal and immune systems; however, from our point of view they are important for the next stages of study of this problem.

In conclusion, inasmuch as the immune reactions represent only one form of the defensive functions of the organism that determine general resistance, the interaction between the hormonal and immune systems cannot be thought of as identical with the influence of hormones on the resistance of the organism. It has been established that the depressive effect of some hormones on the immune response can be correlated with an increase in resistance, and conversely, stimulation of the functions of antibody formation caused by hormonal factors does not always proceed parallel with a rise in general resistance (Astrauskas et al. 1963; Kass 1960). This is due to the varied effect of hormones on different types of protective reactions and the complexity of their interaction with biogenic amines. Therefore the influence of endogenous as well as exogenous hormones on resistance is apparently determined by a complex of their interaction with reactions of specific and nonspecific defense, whose nature may depend on the initial functional state of the corresponding systems at the moment a damaging factor enters the organism, on the intensity of the pathogenic properties of this factor, on the stage of development of the pathological process, and so on. In connection with this, a search for methods of rational therapeutic hormonal intervention in the development of specific pathological states requires further careful study.

6 Organization of the System of Neurohumoral Regulation of Immune Homeostasis
Perspectives and Methods of Investigation (General Conclusions)

The reported data on the possibility of modulating the intensity of immune reactions by acting on various regulatory mechanisms is so extensive and diverse that merely enumerating such influences is not enough to clarify the regulation of the process of immunogenesis.

If all these data are depicted in generalized form (fig. 38), then in evaluating the result of the process—the intensity of antibody production—the neural, hormonal, and mediator factors studied can be classified into three types according to the nature of their action: intensifying factors, suppressing factors, and factors exerting a permissive influence. Even though this scheme does not cover all the factors discovered, in particular the influences of humoral agents, including enzymes, the data already presented need clarification.

Since from the point of view of modern physiology the function of the immune system is visceral, aimed at maintaining the genetic constancy of the cellular composition of the organism—that is, since it is one of the homeostatic mechanisms of the organism as a whole—an attempt to analyze the organization of this function by analogy with other well-studied systems is justified. All the systems studied in physiology follow a common multilevel principle of organization and regulation.

Figure 39 shows the usually observed levels of integration of a system (Chernukh 1976; Laborit 1975), each with its own mechanisms of regulation and autoregulation. Evidently this overall concept holds for the system of immune homeostasis as well, even though its specific mechanisms and interactions are distinctive. For example,

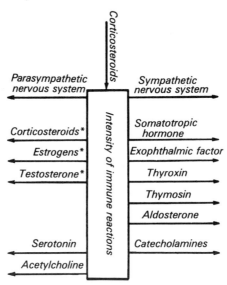

Fig. 38   Factors that alter the intensity of immune reactions. *Arrows pointing up,* stimulation of reactions; *down,* suppression; *horizontal arrow,* permissive influence; *asterisks,* hormones that produce an effect only in large doses.

the high degree of autonomy characteristic of the visceral organs is especially pronounced in this particular case.

As we know, studying the subcellular and cellular mechanisms of regulation of immune processes is the prerogative of biochemists, geneticists, and immunologists. The effect of the steroid hormones of the adrenal glands on the metabolism of the cells of the immune system has been demonstrated, as has the action of adrenergic and noradrenergic substances on these cells. According to one point of view, there are adrenoreceptors and hormone receptors at the surface of the lymph cells. These data suggest that certain nerve impulses originating in adrenergic neurons and certain hormonal (corticosteroid) influences may be aimed directly at the lymph cells. At this cellular level, however, the regulation of the process is determined primarily by the interaction of antigen with the cell and, according to a number of data, by the presence of antibodies that, acting on the cell, bring about regulation by the feedback mechanism.

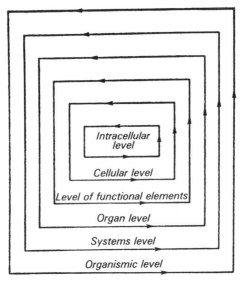

Fig. 39   Hierarchical organization of levels of regulation of functions.
Based on Shkhinek (1975 a, b) and Mountcastle and Powell (1959
a).

Of special interest is the analysis of one of the little-studied levels
of organization—the functional element of an organ. As defined by
Chernukh (1976, 14),

the functional element is a complex microsystem, which includes
the cells and noncellular formations that constitute tissues of an
organ. There are special cells that implement the function of the
functional element, as well as cellular and fibrous components of
the connective tissue. Such structures are arranged around each
microcirculatory unit of an organ, which consists of precapillaries,
capillaries, postcapillary venules, and lymph capillaries. They are
all linked by regulatory mechanisms of physiologically active
substances (including hormones) and neural structures.

The study of the organization of the functions of the immune system
at this level has not yet even begun.

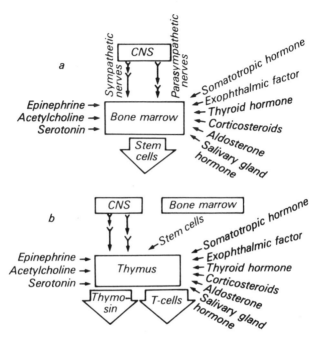

Fig. 40   Complex of factors affecting the functions of the bone marrow (*a*) and the thymus (*b*).

With regard to the regulation of the organs of the lymphatic system, we know they are all equipped with double innervation (fig. 40), but the functional significance of this is practically unknown. In addition, each of the organs of the immune system is under the influence of hormones and other biologically active substances whose significance has been only partly elucidated. For example, the inhibitory effects of corticosteroids on the migration of stem cells have been demonstrated (Plokhinskiy 1970). However, not all of these organs function under equivalent conditions. Thus, when the bone marrow undergoes the influences enumerated above, it produces stem cells, which, upon entering the thymus and the analogue of the bursa of Fabricius, are transformed into T- and B-cells. The function of the thymus thus depends on the number and rate of arrival of stem cells, which are effector elements, but at the same time

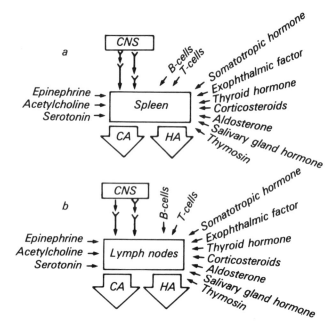

Fig. 41   Complex of factors affecting the functions of the spleen (*a*) and the
lymph nodes (*b*). CA, cellular antibodies; HA, humoral antibodies.

the dynamics of their arrival regulates the activity of the organ (fig. 40*b*).

The spleen and the lymph nodes receive T- and B-dependent lymphocytes, on whose arrival the activity of these organs depends (fig. 41). Thus the organs of the immune system are characterized by the existence of a special and highly important "cellular regulatory channel." The basic relays for the switching from neural and humoral to cellular regulatory mechanisms, that is, the relative importance of the regulatory influences on the functions of the bone marrow, the thymus, and the bursa of Fabricius, deserve special attention.

The systems level of organization of immune homeostasis, which is the primary subject of this book, must be examined with consideration to the neural, endocrine, and other humoral regulatory

mechanisms, their interaction, and their hierarchy. The levels of integration enumerated above are components, whose consolidation into a functionally determined system is brought about by the specific nature of the stimulus—by its antigenicity—with the regulatory mechanisms playing a substantial role in the formation of the whole from the particulars. At present the organization of the system of maintenance of immune homeostasis can still only be tentatively described as a preliminary hypothetical scheme, in which not all the components by far are known or have been studied sufficiently. The regulatory role of the neural and humoral mechanisms boils down to the modulation of immune processes, that is, to changes in their dynamics and intensity. They do not act as triggers, this being the function of antigen action on the cells that bring about immune reactions.

A number of structures in the brain are involved in regulating immune homeostasis—the limbic structures, the hypothalamus, and the reticular formation of the mesencephalon. The involvement of the hypothalamic fields and nuclei and the rearrangement of their mode of operation as they implement the reaction to the antigen, which were demonstrated during the study of the impulse activity of the hypothalamic neurons, indicate, in conjunction with other data, that this region of the brain helps regulate immune reactions under natural conditions. The action of these parts of the CNS on the immunocompetent organs and cells evidently proceeds over various pathways—the sympathetic and parasympathetic nerves going to the lymph organs, the hypophysis, the peripheral endocrine glands, and other humoral paths (fig. 42). The switch from neural to humoral pathways of transmission occurs at the level of hypothalamo-hypophyseal interactions, though it can probably also switch in the lymph organs—by the secretion of mediators at the axon endings of the sympathetic or parasympathetic pathways. In the latter case, the concentration of the appropriate mediators increases in the functional element, and this may lead to a change in microcirculation and in the permeability of the cell membranes, affecting the lymph cells that are capable of responding to the action of a given mediator (e.g., epinephrine or norepinephrine).

Even though the involvement of the endocrine system in the reaction to an antigenic stimulus is far from being fully studied, we can

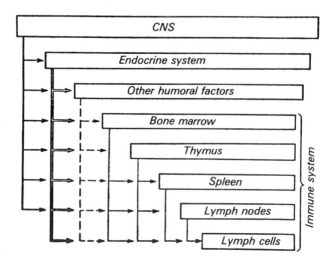

Fig. 42   Possible pathways of regulation of immune homeostasis: neural, endocrine, other humoral and cellular pathways.

assert with regard to the glucocorticoid hormones that the reaction of the adrenal cortex to antigen administration is manifested normally, that it is a stressor reaction, and that it is one of the nonspecific components of the organism's reaction to antigen, the nature and amount of which determine the dynamics of the changes in the corticosteroid level of the blood.

For all the antigens studied, the increase in the 11-hydroxycorticoid level is most pronounced during the first 24 hours after the administration of a foreign protein. As it turned out, the rearrangement observed is rather thorough, since it is also accompanied by a decrease in the amount of bound inactive hormone. The reactions observed depend in large measure on the condition of the central (hypothalamic) regulatory mechanisms: when there is damage to the posterior hypothalamic structures, the intensity of the hormonal response to stressors increases sharply; this does not occur when limited sections of the anterior hypothalamus are destroyed.

At the same time, we do not see a direct dependence of the intensity of the process of antibody production on hormonal reactions of this kind, even though the glucocorticoids are known to affect me-

tabolism in the lymph cells and the migration of stem cells and thymus cells. It is possible that in the intact organism the corticosteroids participate in implementing only certain stages of the immune process and that, being essential components, they act permissively in physiological doses. As was shown in the experiments of E. K. Shkhinek, K. Szalai, and K. Abavári (unpublished data), in the case of intravenous immunization the primary immune response may also develop against the background of a decrease in the amount of mineralocorticoids (aldosterone) in the blood; that is, under certain conditions the reactions of the glucocorticoid and mineralocorticoid hormones may be opposite. The functional significance of this combination requires further experimental study. Apparently the hormonal background that develops when foreign proteins enter the internal environment of the organism is sufficiently complex and significant, specifically in certain types of combinations of various hormonal and other humoral components of the process. The relative significance of these components is a promising subject for further research.

One of the most important problems of the regulation of immune homeostasis concerns the mechanisms that control input of information about foreign protein into the CNS. It appears logical to assume a humoral and, probably, mediated means of transmission of this kind of information and the immunologic nonspecificity of the information. The resources of modern physiology and immunology will permit a study of this problem in the near future, though at present the procedural difficulties are obvious, as they are in the analysis of the pathways of reverse afferentation (feedback) at different hierarchical levels of the process.

Since the maintenance of immune homeostasis is a multicomponent process, its study is particularly difficult, but it is clear that it is essential to determine the possible cycle of regulatory influences on each component of the process and on their interaction. The relative importance of regulatory (neurohumoral) factors in the intensity of the immune response or function of the immunocompetent organs, that is, the relation between genetically predetermined types of response and those determined by the specific situation of the organism and the environment, remains a fundamental problem.

On the basis of the data obtained thus far, it is evident that, in the dynamics of the immune process, some phases or components are particularly sensitive to various regulatory factors and their complexes. This creates considerable difficulties in studying the operation of the system as a whole, since we are dealing with a multicomponent system, multichannel efferent pathways, and the nonsynchronous interaction of regulatory and effector elements. Constructing a model of this interaction that is close to reality will probably become possible only with the use of mathematical methods of analysis and computer technology (Chubukhchiyev et al. 1976). The input of large amounts of information that is basically uniform but has been obtained in different experimental variants can reveal the most general principles of the process. However, to develop a realistic model of the process it is necessary to analyze strictly comparable results, obtained for animals of the same genetic line, with the use of the same antigen, and then correlate them with data obtained by the same method but on different animals, with different proteins, so as to determine the general and specific principles of the regulation of immune homeostasis.

The study of the neurohumoral regulation of immune homeostasis as a branch of modern physiology has developed during the past decade; it has taken the first tangible steps in experimental research, has already drawn together a large international group of scientists, and holds promise in regard to the analysis of the activity of the immune system as one of the functions of the organism aimed at maintaining the constancy of its internal environment.

Epilogue

Since the Russian edition of our book was published, several new developments have taken place. Among these I should mention two in particular:

1. The discovery of neuromediator and hormonal receptors on the membranes of lymphoid cells (Hadden et al. 1970; Weinstein and Melmon 1976; Gordon et al. 1978, Delespesse et al. 1980).

2. The demonstration that secondary messengers (cyclic nucleotides) participate in information transfer from the surfaces of cells to intracellular structures and in the metabolism and functional activity of lymphocytes. Such research has made it possible to elucidate at least in part the nature of the biological molecular basis for the interaction between the neural, endocrine, and immune systems on lymphoid cells (Korneva 1982; Poltavchenko 1982; Shkhinek et al. 1982 a,b). A major achievement in immunophysiology is represented by investigations of the role of humoral factors of bone marrow in the regulating functions of the immune system. Major contributions in this area were made by Pierpaoli (1981), Maestroni et al. (1982), Mikhaylova (1981), and Petrov et al. (1981).

In May 1982 a symposium was organized in Leningrad on problems of regulation of immune homeostasis. This symposium was attended by scientists from the Soviet Union, Argentina, Hungary, the United States, Switzerland, and Yugoslavia, indicating an increasing interest in this problem. The early beginnings of these investigations go back to the start of this century and are connected with such names as I. G. Savchenko, A. Metal'nikov, and A. D. Speranskiy.

168

New developments in this field have been stimulated by the work of clinicians, physiologists, and neurologists.

Clinicians have observed in patients with neuropsychiatric disorders changes in immune status and in the ability to resist infectious diseases. Conversely, physicians have observed that disturbances in immune reactions may lead to various disorders of the nervous system. Physiologists became involved in research on immune processes because they realized there must be an interrelation between the functions of the immune system in the intact organism and the endocrine and neural systems. Immunologists began to realize that there must be a difference between in vitro experiments and what may take place in the organism as a whole. Thus it became obvious that it is necessary to investigate how various regulatory systems contribute to the development and maintenance of immune homeostasis. As a result of the cooperation between clinicians, physiologists, and immunologists, a new discipline developed that is referred to as immunophysiology. The object of immunophysiology is to investigate physiological mechanisms underlying the regulation of immune processes in the intact organism, utilizing physiological, immunologic, and biochemical methods, and thus to gain knowledge about the possibilities of influencing the immune processes in relation to health maintenance.

Overall, modern medicine has at its disposal several agents that may influence the course of infectious disorders. These include antibiotics, sulfonamides, and vaccines. However, thus far we have very little knowledge about the nature of immune processes and the mechanisms the body uses in developing resistance to diseases. The task of immunophysiology is to learn about the nature of immune processes in the intact organism and to discover something about the possibilities of influencing the organism's resistance to diseases. The distinguished Soviet neurophysiologist N. P. Bekhtereva referred to regulation of immune homeostasis as a most important problem in physiology, since it deals not only with mechanisms involved in resistance to infectious diseases, but also with such areas as oncology, genetic defects, and so forth.

Since our publication on the participation of subcortical components of the central nervous system in immune homeostasis (Korneva and Khay 1963), numerous studies have appeared regarding

the influence of various structures of the CNS on the immune system. Data have been published on participation by the posterior regions of the hypothalamus, by other components of the hypothalamus, by the limbic system, and by the hippocampus in the regulation of cellular and humoral immunity and autoimmune processes (Leonavichene 1981; Korneva 1982; Polyak et al. 1982). Shekoyan (1977) and Korneva and Shekoyan (1982) reported that destroying hypothalamic structures led to changes in the functional activity of the system of macrophagal phagocytosis. Some studies have shown that changes in the activity of structures of the dorsal hippocampus elicited by local stimulation or destruction of the structures led to an immunodeficient condition characterized by disturbances in immune functions and nonspecific resistance to infectious diseases (see S. V. Magayeva 1979). Klimenko (1981) demonstrated significant changes in neurophysiological functioning in hypothalamic structures after immunization. He demonstrated differences in changes in functional activity in the hypothalamic structures following primary, as contrasted with secondary, immune responses. He also reported that, following immunization, he observed periods of increased excitabililty in the amygdala comparable to those he recorded in the posterior hypothalamus.

Grigor'yev (1982) described definite patterns of inclusion of various nuclear formations in the hypothalamus in response to antigenic stimulation, suggesting a definite sequential order of inclusion of various parts of this neurophysiologic system in the course of immune reactions. Valuyeva et al. (1982) and Kozlov (1980) reported on the significant roles played by the hormones of the thymus, hypophysis, adrenal cortex, and thyroid and parathyroid glands in processes of migration, proliferation, and differentiation of different groups of lymphoid cells, thus delineating their role in the development of cellular and humoral immune reactions to the actions of these humoral endogenous stimuli.

Shkhinek et al. (1982 a,b) reported on changes in the mineralocorticoid functions of the hypothalamohypophysio-adrenocortical system (HHAS) soon after introduction of antigens into the body. Trufakin et al. (1977) reported that administering somatotropin prevented the development of autoimmune reactions. Shekoyan et al. (1982) reported that hypofunction of the parathyroid glands de-

creased immune reactions. He also described the role of macrophages in the mechanisms of action of parathyroid hormones on the course of immune reactions. Fedoseyev et al. (1982) and Golubeva et al. (1979, 1982) reported on immunostimulating effects of amphetamine and immunoblocking effects of the alpha-adrenergic blocking agent phenoxybenzamine. Gordon et al. (1982) reported on changes in the level and distribution of biogenic amines in lymphoid organs following the administration of antigens. Devoyno and Al'perina (1982) demonstrated the participation of the serotonergic system on immunogenesis: an inhibiting effect via the adrenal glands and a stimulating effect via the thymus.

More research is needed to elucidate the mechanisms involved in interactions between hormones in the immune system and in their interactions with the nervous system. In particular, more direct data are needed on afferent pathways and mechanisms of information processing in the nervous system after antigens are introduced into the organism.

Elena A. Korneva

1983

References

Abinder, A. A. 1963. Vliyaniye izmenennogo sostoyaniya tsentral'noy nervnoy sistemy na perestroyku immunogennoy reaktivnosti organizma i techeniye anafilakticheskogo shoka (The influence of the altered state of the central nervous system on the change in the reactivity of the organism and the course of anaphylactic shock). *Zhur. Mikrobiol., Epidemiol., Immunobiol.* 34 (10):17-21.

Ablin, R. J.; Bruns, G. R.; Guinau, P.; and Bush, J. M. 1974a. Antiandrogenic suppression of lymphocytic blastogenesis: In vitro and in vivo observations. *Experientia* 30:1351-53.

———. 1974b. The effect of oestrogen on the incorporation of H^3-timidine by PHA-stimulated human peripheral blood lymphocytes. *J. Immunol.* 113:705-7.

Ach, Zs.; Stark, E.; and Csaki, L. 1967. The effect of long-term corticotrophin treatment of the corticosteroid binding capacity of transcortin. *J. Endocrinol.* 39:565-69.

Adam, J., and Enke, H. 1970. Zur Anwendung der Faktorenanalyse als Trennverfahren. *Biometr. Z.* 12:395-411.

Adamov, A. K., and Nikolayev, N. I. 1968. *Molekulyarno-kletochnyye osnovy immunologii* (Molecular and cellular principles of immunology). Saratov.

Ader, Robert, ed. 1981. *Psychoneuroimmunology.* New York: Academic Press.

Adler, F. L.; Fishman, M.; and Dray, S. 1966. Antibody formation initiated in vitro. 3. Antibody formation and allotypic specificity directed by ribonucleic acid and from peritoneal exudate cells. *J. Immunol.* 97:554.

Ado, A. D. 1952. *Antigeny kak chrezvychaynyye razdrazhiteli nervnoy sistemy* (Antigens as extraordinary stimulants of the nervous system). Moscow.

_____. 1957. O mekhanizmakh deystviya mikrobov i virusov na nervnuyu sistemu (The mechanism of action of microbes and viruses on the nervous system). In *O mekhanizmakh deystviya mikrobov na nervnuyu sistemu* (Mechanisms of the action of microbes on the nervous system), 3–17. Moscow.

_____. 1959. O patofiziologicheskikh mekhanizmakh immuniteta (Pathophysiological mechanisms of immunity). In *Doklady XIII Vsesoyuznogo s"ezda gigiyenistov, epidemiologov, mikrobiologov i infektsionistov* (Proceedings of the thirteenth all-Union congress of hygienists, epidemiologists, microbiologists, and infectionists), 2:110–13. Moscow.

Ado, A. D., and Gol'dshteyn, M. M. 1974. Yavlyayutsya li zadniye otdely gipotalamusa "gipotalamicheskimi tsentrami regulyatsii immunogeneza"? (Are the posterior sections of the hypothalamus "hypothalamic centers for the regulation of immunogenesis"?). *Fiziol. Zhurn. SSSR* 60(4):548–55.

Ado, A. D., and Gushchin, I. S. 1965. Vliyaniye povrezhdeniya ventromedial'noy oblasti srednego gipotalamusa na chuvstvitel'nost' belykh krys k yaichnomu belku (The influence of damage to the ventromedial section of the middle hypothalmus on the sensitivity of white rats to ovalabumin). In *Mater. Vsesoyuzn. konf. "fiziologiya i patologiya gipotalamusa"* (Proceedings of the all-Union conference on physiology and pathology of the hypothalamus), 7–8. Moscow.

Ado, A. D., and Ishimova, L. M. 1958. K voprosu o reflektornom mekhanizme obrazovaniya antitel (On the reflex mechanism of antibody formation). *Byull. Eksp. Biol. Med.* 46(11):22–27.

Ado, A. D., and Kibyakov, A. V. 1941. Cited in Kozlov (1968).

Aleshin, B. V. 1971. *Gistofiziologiya gipotalamo-gipofizarnoy sistemy* (Histophysiology of the hypothalamohypophyseal system). Moscow.

Alifanov, V. V.; Moiseyenko, Ye. A.; Tomich, M. A.; Shul'govskiy, V. V.; and Kotlyar, B. I. 1968. Nekotoryye rezul'taty obrabotki impul'snoy aktivnosti neyronov s pomoshch'yu statisticheskikh metodov (Some results of the treatment of the pulse activity of neurons with the aid of statistical methods). In *Statisticheskaya elektrofiziologiya*, ch. 1 (Statistical electrophysiology, part 1), 26–34. Vilnius.

Al'pern, D. Ye. 1964. Gipotalamo-gipofizarno-adrenalovaya sistema v patogeneze allergii (The hypothalamohypophophysio-adrenal system in the pathogenesis of allergy). In *Gipofiz-kora nadpochechnikov* (Hypophysioadrenal cortex), 72–78. Kiev.

Ambrose, C. T. 1964. The requirement for hydrocortisone in antibody-forming tissue cultivated in serum-free medium. *J. Exp. Med.* 119:1027–49.

_____. 1966. Biochemical agents affecting the inductive phase of the secondary antibody response initiated in vitro. *Bacteriol. Rev.* 30:408–17.

_____. 1970. The essential role of corticosteroids in the induction of immune response in vitro. In *Hormones and the immune response*, ed. G. E. W. Wolstenholme and J. Knight, 1–116. London: Churchill.

Ambrose, C. T., and Coons, A. H. 1963. The replacement of serum by hydrocortisone in the production of antibody in vitro. *Fed. Proc.* 22(1):266.

Amkraut, A. A., and Solomon, G. F. 1975. From the symbolic stimulus to the pathophysiologic response: Immune mechanisms. *Int. J. Psych. Med.* 5:541–63.

Anand, B. K., and Pillai, P. V. 1967. Activity of single neurones in the hypothalamic feeding centres: Effect of gastric distension. *J. Physiol.* 192:63–77.

Anand, B. K.; Chhina, G. S.; and Singh, B. 1962. Effect of glucose on the activity of hypothalamic "feeding centres." *Science* 138:597–98.

Anand, B. K.; Banerjee, M. C.; and Chhina, G. S. 1966. Single neurone; activity of hypothalamic feeding centres: Effect of local heating. *Brain Res.* 1:269–78.

Andersen, P. 1964. The role in the phasing of spontaneous thalamocortical discharge. *J. Physiol.* 173:459–80.

Andersen, P., and Eccles, J. C. 1962. Inhibitory phasing of neuronal discharge. *Nature* 196:645–47.

Andersson, B., and Blomgren, H. 1970. Evidence for a small pool of immunocompetent cells in the mouse thymus: Its role in the humoral antibody response against sheep erythrocytes, bovine serum albumin, ovalbumin, and NIP determinant. *Cell Immunol.* 1:362–71.

_____. 1971. Evidence for thymus-independent humoral antibody production in mice against polyvinylpyrrolidone and E. coli lipopolysaccharide. *Cell Immunol.* 2:411–16.

Anokhin, P. K. 1957. Znacheniye retikulyarnoy formatsii dlya razlichnykh form vysshey nervnoy deyatel'nosti (The significance of the reticular formation for various forms of higher nervous activity). *Fiziol. Zh. SSSR* 43(11):1072–85.

Anokhin, P. K., and Sudakov, K. V. 1970. Neyrofiziologicheskiye mekhanizmy goloda i nasyshcheniya (Neurophysiological mechanisms of hunger and saturation). In *Materialya XI s"ezda Vsesoyuznogo fiziologicheskogo obshchestva imeni I. P. Pavlova* (Proceedings of the eleventh congress of the I. P. Pavlov all-Union physiological society), 284–89. Leningrad.

Antonichev, A. V., and Rozen, V. B. 1967. Znacheniye gipofiza v svyazyvanii gidrokortizona plazmy kortikoidsvyazyvayushchim globulinom u

morskikh svinok (The significance of the hypophysis in the fixation of the plasma hydrocortisone by corticoid-fixing globulin in guinea pigs). *Probl. Endokrinol.* 13(6):85–88.

Arend, Yu. O. 1963. O vliyanii povrezhdeniya gipotalamicheskoy oblasti na proliferativnyye protsessy soyedinitel'noy tkani u krolikov (The influence of damage to the hypothalamic region on the proliferation processes of the connective tissue in rabbits). *Tr. Po Meditsine Tartuskogo Gos. Unta* (Tartu State Univ. Med. Publications) 8(143):300–303.

Ass-Babich, B. T. 1966. Vliyaniye tireoidektomii na dinamiku plazmotsitarnoy reaktsii i serologicheskikh sdvigov pri immunizatsii protiv bryushnogo tifa (The influence of thyroidectomy on the dynamics of the plasmocyte reaction and serological changes upon immunization against typhus abdominalis). In *Voprosy immunologii* (Problems of immunology), 2:21–25. Kiev.

Astaf'yeva, N. G. 1970. O roli gipotalamo-gipofizarno-nadpochechnikovoy sistemy v mekhanizme razvitiya demiyeliniziruyushchikh zabolevaniy (na modeli eksperimental'nogo allergicheskogo entsefalomiyelita) Avtoref. kand. dis. (The role of the hypothalamohypophsio-adrenal system in the mechanism of the development of demyelinizing diseases, modeled by experimental allergic encephalomyelitis. Dissertation), Saratov.

Astrauskas, V. I. 1968. Gipotalamo-gipofizarno-nadpochechnikovaya sistema i reaktivnost' organizma (The hypothalamohypophysio-adrenal system and the reactivity of the organism. Dissertation). Vilnius.

Astrauskas, V. I., and Leonavichene, L. K. 1975. Vliyaniye proizvodnogo oksialkilamidov dikarbonovykh kislot na bioelektricheskuyu aktivnost' obrazovaniy golovnogo mozga i immunnyye reaktsii pri eksperimental'-'nom revmaticheskom protsesse u krolikov s koagulirovannymi zadnegipotalamicheskimi yadrami (The influence of the derivative of oxyalkylamides of dicarboxylic acids on the bioelectric activity of formations of the brain and immune reactions in an experimental rheumatic process in rabbits with coagulated posterohypothalamic nuclei. In *Neyrogumoral'naya i farmakologicheskaya korrektsiya immunologicheskikh reaktsiy v eksperimente i klinike. Tez. dokl.* (Neurohumoral and pharmacologic correction of immune reactions under experimental and clinical conditions. Proceedings), 5–6. Leningrad.

Astrauskas, V. I.; Mishkinite, G. I.; Sbichulis, A. K.; Krasnodomskens, A. I.; and Lyatukems, Ye. V. 1963. Znacheniye gipofizarno-adrenalovoy sistemy dlya razvitiya protsessov sensibilizatsii (The significance of the hypophysio-adrenal system in the development of sensitization processes). In *Voprosy immunopatologii* (Problems of immunopathology), 208–10. Moscow.

Asyamolova, I. A. 1958. Vliyaniye aminazina na vegetativnyye uslovnyye refleksy i EEG u desimpatizirovannykh i intaktnykh krolikov (The influence of chlorpromazine on vegetative conditioned reflexes and the electroencephalogram in desympathectomized and intact rabbits). In *Vliyaniye aminazina na TsNS. Tez. dokl. nauchn. konf.* (The influence of chlorpromazine on the central nervous system. Proceedings of the scientifiic conference), 4–5. Leningrad.

Aver'yanova, L. L. 1970. Nervnodistroficheskiy komponent v razvitii eksperimental'nogo endomiokardita (The neurodystrophic component in the development of experimental endomyocarditis). In *Nervnaya trofika v fiziologii i patologii* (Nervous trophism in physiology and pathology), 198–207. Moscow.

Avetikyan, B. G., and Melkumyan, M. A. 1956a. O roli nervnoy sistemy v immunologicheskikh reaktsiyakh (The role of the nervous system in immune reactions). *Zhurn, Mikrobiol., Epidemiol., Immunobiol.* 26(5):53–54.

———. 1956b. O vliyanii fenamina na agglyutinatsionnyy titr syvorotki immunizirovannykh zhivotnykh (On the influence of amphetamine on the agglutination titer of serum of immunized animals). In *Osnovy immuniteta* (Principles of immunity), 118–25. Moscow.

Azhipa, Ya. I. 1976. *Nervy zhelez vnutrenney sekretsii i mediatory v regulyatsii endokrinnykh funktsiy* (The nerves of the endocrine glands and mediators in the regulation of endocrine functions). Moscow.

Bach, J. F., and Dardenne, M. 1971. Cited in Uteshev and Babichev (1974).

Baklavadzhan, O. G. 1969. Gipotalamus (The hypothalamus). In *Obshchaya i chastnaya fiziologiya nervnoy sistemy* (General and particular physiology of the nervous system), 362–87. Leningrad.

Balabolkin, M. I. 1971. *Somatotropnyy gormon peredney doli gipofiza* (The somatotropic hormone of the anterior lobe of the hypophysis). Moscow.

Balow, J. E.; Hurley, D. L.; and Fauce, A. S. 1975. Immunosuppressive effects of glucocorticoids: Differential effects of acute VS chronic administration of cell mediated immunity. *J. Immunol.* 114:1072–76.

Baroni, C. 1967. Thymus, peripheral lymphoid tissues and immunological responsiveness of the pituitary dwarf mouse. *Experientia* 23:282–83.

Baroni, C.; Fabris, N.; and Bertoli, G. 1967. Age dependence of the primary immune response in the hereditary pituitary and hormonal Snell-Bagg mouse. *Experientia* 23:1059–60.

Barraclough, C. A., and Cross, B. A. 1963. Unit activity in the hypothalamus of the cyclic female rat: Effect of genital stimuli and progesterone. *J. Endocrinol.* 26:339–59.

Baust, W., and Katz, P. 1961. Untersuchungen zur tonisierung einzelner Neurone im hinteren Hypothalamus. *Pflüg. Arch.* 272:575–90.

Baydakov, P. A. 1958. Vliyaniye anafilaksii na uslovnoreflektornuyu deyatel'nost' zhivotnykh (krolikov) (The influence of anaphylaxis on the conditioned reflex activity of animals [rabbits]). *Tr. Voronezhskogo Med. Inta* (Proceedings of the Voronezh Medical Institute), 30:85–90.

Bedretdinov, Kh. A.; Berlin, A. N.; Filippov, G. I.; and Yatsevich, V. V. 1969. *Faktornyy i komponentnyy analiz* (Factor and component analysis). Moscow.

Bekhtereva. N. P.; Bundzen, P. V.; Matveyev, Yu. K.; and Kaplunovskiy, A. S. 1971. Funktsional'naya reorganizatsiya aktivnosti neyronnykh populyatsiy mozga cheloveka pri kratkovremennoy verbal'noy pamyati (Functional reorganization of the activity of the human brain in short-term verbal memory). *Fiziol. Zh. SSSR* 57(12):1745–61.

Belasic, M.; Grebacova, J.; and Mjartanova, J. 1956. Vztah intenzity tuberkulinovych reakcii k tonusu a dráždivosti vegetatívného nervstva (The relation between the intensity of tuberculin reactions to the tonus and the excitability of the vegetative nervous system). *Bratisl. Lekar. Listy* 1:331–39.

Belen'kiy, G. S. 1955. K voprosu o fiziologicheskom mekhanizme kortikal'noy regulyatsii sostava perifericheskoy krovi (On the physiological mechanism of cortical regulation of the composition of the peripheral blood). *Fiziol. Zhurn. SSSR* 41(6):765–69.

Beling, C. C., and Weksler, M. E. 1974. Suppression of mixed lymphocyte reactivity by human chorionic gonadotrophin. *Clin. Exptl. Immunol.* 18:537–41.

Belovolova, R. A. 1973. Nekotoryye aspekty neyrogumoral'noy regulyatsii immunogeneza. Avtoref. kand. dis. (Some aspects of neurohumoral regulation of immunogenesis. Dissertation). Rostov-on-Don.

Belyavskiy, A. D. 1958. Rol' TsNS v razvitii fagotsitarnoy reaktsii (The role of the central nervous system in the development of the phagocytic reaction). In *Studencheskiye raboty Rostovskogo Meditsinskogo Instituta* (Students' works of the Rostov-on-Don Medical Institute), 1:55–56.

Belyavskiy, Ye. M. 1966. Vliyaniye pirogenov na temperaturnuyu chuvstvitel'nost' perednego gipotalamusa (The influence of pyrogens on the temperature sensitivity of the anterior hypothalamus. Dissertation). Leningrad.

————. 1974. Izmeneniye aktivnosti termochuvstvitel'nykh neyronov perednego gipotalamusa pod vliyaniyem pirogenov (The change in the activity of thermosensitive neurons of the anterior hypothalamus under the influence of pyrogens). In *Teoreticheskiye i prakticheskiye voprosy*

termoregulyatsii v norme i patologii. Tez. konf. (Theoretical and practical problems of thermoregulation under normal and pathologic conditions. Proceedings of the conference), 40–41. Leningrad.

Benetato, Gr. 1952. Rolul sistemului nervos central in procesele immunobiologice (The role of the central nervous system in immunobiologic processes). *Revista Stiintelor Medicale: Medicina Interna.* 9:21–24.

———. 1955. Le mécanisme nerveux central de la réaction leucocytaire et phagocytaire. *J. Physiol.* (Paris) 47:391–403.

Benetato, Gr.; Bacin, J.; and Vlad, L. 1945. Zentralnervensystem und Abwehrfunktion. *Schweiz. Med. Wschr.* 75:702–4.

Benetato, Gr.; Bajuku, U.; and Kukujanu, M. 1958. O roli nadpochechnikov v podderzhanii belkovogo sostava krovi i v obrazovanii antitel (The role of the adrenal glands in the maintenance of the protein composition of the blood and in antibody formation). *Patol. Fiziol. Eksperim. Terap.* 2(5):11–16.

Bennett, M., and Cudkowich, Z. L. 1968. Hemopoietic progenitor cells with limited potential for differentiation: Erythropoietic function of mouse marrow "lymphocytes." *J. Cell Physiol.* 72:129.

Berger, M.; Strecker, H. J.; and Waelsch, H. 1956. Action of chlorpromazine on oxidative phosphorylation of liver and brain mitochondria. *Nature* 177: 1234–35.

Berglund, K. 1956a. Studies on factors which condition the effect of cortisone on antibody production. 2. The significance of the dose of antigen in primary hemolysin response. *Acta Path. Mikrobiol. Scand.* 38:329–38.

———. 1956b. Studies on factors which condition the effect of cortisone on antibody production. 4. The significance of the particle size of the antigen. *Acta Path. Microbiol. Scand.* 39:41–46.

Berglund, K., and Fagraens, A. 1961. Studies on the antibody-formation in cortisone treated rats. *Acta Path. Microbiol. Scand.* 52:321–29.

Beritov, I. S. 1950. O proiskhozhdenii spontannoy aktivnosti i peredache vozbuzhdeniya v nervnykh uzlakh bryushnoy tsepochki piyavki (The origin of spontaneous activity and transfer of excitation in the nerve ganglia of the abdominal chain of the leech). *Zh. Obshch. Biol.* 9:31.

———. 1959. *Obshchaya fiziologiya myshechnoy i nervnoy systemy* (General physiology of the muscular and nervous system), vol. 2. Moscow.

Bernasconi, C.; Lazzarino, M.; Pontigia, P.; and Introzzi, A. M. 1967. Cited in Uteshev and Babichev (1974).

Bernett, F. 1971. *Kletochnaya immunologiya* (Cellular immunology). Moscow.

Bilenko, V. I.; Bogdanova, V. L.; and Tseytlik, V. L. 1975. Limfotsitotoksicheskiy effekt prednizolona i purinovykh antimetabolitov na razlich-

nyye vidy limfotsitov intaktnykh sobak i sobak s allotransplantirovannoy pochkoy (The lymphocytotoxic effect of prednisolone and purine antimetabolites on various types of lymphocytes of intact dogs and dogs with allotransplanted kidneys). In *Neyrogumoral'naya i farmakologicheskaya korrektsiya immunologicheskoy reaktsii v eksperimente i klinike.* Tez. dokl. (Neurohumoral and pharmacologic correction of immune reaction under experimental and clinical conditions. Proceedings), 6–7. Leningrad.

Biornbol, Fischel, and Stark. 1951. Cited in Zdrodovskiy (1969).

Biryukov, D. A. 1958. K voprosu o topike deystviya aminazina (The problem of localization of action of chlorpromazine). In *Vliyaniye aminazina na TsNS.* Tez. dokl. (The influence of chlorpromazine on the central nervous system. Proceedings), 7–8. Leningrad.

Blomgren, H. 1971. Studies on the proliferation of thymus cells injected into syngeneic or allogeneic irradiated mice. *Clin. Exp. Immunol.* 8:279–89.

Bogdanchikova, V. V. 1968. K voprosu o roli gipotalamicheskoy oblasti v formirovanii nekotorykh immunologicheskikh reaktsiy (On the question of the role of the hypothalamic area in the development of certain immune reactions. Dissertation). Donetsk.

Bogendorfer, L. 1927. Über den Einfluss des Zentralnervensystems auf Immunitätsvorgänge. 2. Mitt. *Arch. Exp. Pharmacol.* 24:378–80.

Bondarev, I. M. 1963. *Patogenez eksperimental'noy tuberkuleznoy kaverny legkogo u sobak* (Pathogenesis of experimental tuberculous pulmonary cavern in dogs. Dissertation). Rostov-on-Don.

_____. 1967. Usvoyeniye razdrazheniya—osnovnoye usloviye vozniknoveniya tuberkuleznoy kaverny legkogo (Assimilation of the stimulus—the basic condition for the genesis of a tuberculous cavern of the lung). In *Patogenez i samogenez ochagovykh i destruktivnykh form tuberkuleza* (Pathogenesis and autogenesis of focal and destructive forms of tuberculosis), 66–70. Moscow.

Bonvallet, M.; Dell, P.; and Hiebel, J. 1954. Tonus sympathique et activité électrique corticale. *EEG Clin. Neurophysiol.* 6:119–44.

Bösing-Scheider, R. 1975. Differential effects of cyclic AMP on the in vitro induction of antibody synthesis. *Nature* 256:137–38.

Braun, W. 1973. Role of cyclic nucleotides in the regulation of immune responses. In *Prostaglandins and cyclic AMP biological actions and clinical application,* 227–28. New York.

Braun, W., and Ishizuka, M. 1971. Cyclic AMP and immune responses. 2. Phospodiesterase inhibitors as potentiators of polynucleotide effects on antibody formation. *J. Immunol.* 107:1036–42.

Brighenti, L., and Gioelli, A. 1966. Cited in Uteshev and Babichev (1974).

Brooks, C. M. C. 1959. Electrical activity of the ventromedial nuclei of the hypothalamus. *Amer. J. Physiol.* 197:829.

Broun, G. R. 1969a. Issledovaniye funktsional'nogo sostoyaniya medial' nykh struktur srednego gipotalamusa pri eksperimental'nom tuberkuleze (Investigation of the functional state of the medial structures of the middle hypothalamus in experimental tuberculosis). *Patol. Fiziol. I Eksper. Terap.* 13(1):73–74.

———. 1969b. K kharakteristike funktsional'nogo sostoyaniya nekotorykh struktur gipotalamusa pri eksperimental'nom tuberkuleze (Characteristics of the functional state of the hypothalamus in experimental tuberculosis. Dissertation). Leningrad.

Brown, G. M., and Reichlin, S. 1972. Psychologic and neural regulation of growth hormone secretion. *Psychosom. Med.* 34:45–61.

Budylin, N. V. 1953. K voprosu o vliyanii tsentral'noy nervnoy sistemy na obrazovaniye immuntel (On the question of the influence of the central nervous system on the formation of immune bodies). *Zhurn. Mikrobiol., Epidemiol., Immunobiol.* 9:53–63.

Bundzen, P. V.; Vasilevskiy, N. N.; Kaplunovskiy, A. S.; and Shabayev, V. V. 1971. Primeneniye faktornogo analiza dlya izucheniya funktsional'noy organizatsii dinamicheskikh kharakteristik bioelektricheskoy aktivnosti golovnog o mozga (The application of factor analysis for the study of the functional organization of the dynamic characteristics of the bioelectric activity of the brain). *Fiziol. Zhurn. SSSR* 57(6):969.

Burns, B. D.; Heron, W.; and Pritchard, R. 1962. Physiological excitation of visual cortex in cats' unanaesthetized isolated forebrain. *J. Neurophysiol.* 25:165.

Burykina, G. N., and Krylov, S. S. 1975. Narusheniye funktsiy gipotalamo-gipofizarnoy sistemy v patogeneze allergicheskikh dermatozov i vozmozhnosti lekarstvennoy terapii (Disturbance of the functions of the hypothalamohypophyseal system in the pathogenesis of allergic dermatoses and possibilities of medicinal therapy). In *Neyrogumoral'naya farmakologicheskiya korrektsiya immunologicheskikh reaktsiy v eksperimente i klinike.* Tez. dokl. (Neurohumoral and pharmacologic correction of immune reactions under experimental and clinical conditions. Proceedings), 7–8. Leningrad.

Buss, K., and Buss, H. 1970. Bioloģisko objektu klasifikācija ar komponent-analīzi (The classification of biological objects by means of component analysis). *Jaunāk. Mežsaimniecībā* 13:3–7.

Buyanskaya, M. D. 1952. K voprosu o vliyanii nervnoy sistemy na immunitet. 1. Vliyaniye adrenalina, atropina i pilokarpina na vyrabotku antitel

(On the question of the influence of the nervous system on immunity. 1. The influence of epinephrine, atropine, and pilocarpine on antibody production). *Tr. Ivanovskogo Med. In-ta* (Proceedings of the Ivanovo Med. Inst.), 8:67–76.

Cabanac, M.; Stolwijk, J. A. J.; and Hardy, J. D. 1968. Effect of temperature and pyrogens on single-unit activity in the rabbit's brain stem. *J. Appl. Physiol.* 24:645–52.

Cannon, W. B. 1929. *Bodily changes in pain, hunger, fear and rage.* New York.

Castro, J. E. 1973. Androgen deprivation as a stimulant of immunity. In *Non-specific factors influencing host resistance,* 277–84. Basel.

————. 1974. Orchidectomy and the immune response. 1. Effect of orchidectomy on lymphoid tissues of mice. *Proc. Roy. Soc.* (London) 185:425–36.

Chaplinskiy, V. Ya. 1973. Fazovyye izmeneniya immunologicheskoy reaktivnosti gipotireoidnykh krolikov v zavisimosti ot vremeni, proshedshego posle vyklyucheniya deyatel'nosti shchitovidnoy zhelezy (Phase changes in immune reactivity of hypothyroid rabbits in relation to the time passed after elimination of the activity of the thyroid gland). In *Immunologiya* (Immunology), 6:19–21. Kiev.

Char, D. F. B., and Kelley, V. C. 1962. Serum antibody and protein studies following adrenalectomy in rabbits. *Proc. Soc. Exp. Biol. Med.* 109:599–602.

Chebotarev, V. R. 1965. Sravnitel'naya kharakteristika nekotorykh immunobiologicheskikh pokazateley pri vvedenii gidrokortizona i dezoksikortikosteron-atsetata (Comparative characteristics of certain immunobiological indicators upon administration of hydrocortisone and deoxycorticosterone acetate). In *Voprosy immunologii* (Problems of immunology), 48–52. Kiev.

————. 1966. Izucheniye plazmokletochnoy reaktsii limfaticheskikh uzlov krys pri immunizatsii s primeneniyem gidrokortizona i dezoksikortikosterona (DOKSA) (The study of the plasmocellular reaction of the lymph nodes of rats upon immunization with the application of hydrocortisone and deoxycorticosterone (DOCA). In *Voprosy immunologii* (Problems of immunology), 2:16–20. Kiev.

Chebotarev, V. R., and Valuyeva, T. K. 1972. Vliyaniye adrenalektomii na formirovaniye antiteloobrazuyushchikh kletok u zhivotnykh s giperchuvstvitel'nost'yu zamedlennogo tipa (The influence of adrenalectomy on the development of antibody-forming cells in animals with hypersensitivity of the delayed type). *Zhurn. Mikrobiol., Epidemiol., Immunobiol.* 42(10):128–31.

Chernigovskaya, N. V.; Korneva, Ye. A.; Konovalov, G. V.; and Khay,

L. M. 1975. Mezodientsefal'nyye struktury mozga v patogeneze demiyeliniziruyushchikh zabolevaniy nervnoy sistemy (Mesodiencephalic structures of the brain in the pathogenesis of demyelinizing diseases of the nervous system). In *Demiyeliniziruyushchiye zabolevaniya nervnoy sistemy
v eksperimente i klinike* (Demyelinizing diseases of the nervous system
under experimental and clinical conditions), 226–334. Minsk.

Chernukh, A. M. 1976. Funktsional'nyy element-organ-organizm (Functional element-organ-organism). In *Mekhanizmy povrezhdeniya, rezistentnosti, adaptatsii i kompensatsii. Tez. dokl.* (Mechanisms of injury,
resistance, adaptation, and compensation. Proceedings), 1:13–17. Tashkent.

Chernukh, A. M., and Tolmacheva, N. S. 1963. K voprosu ob izuchenii
mekhanizmov vyzdorovleniya i eksperimental'noy terapii allergicheskikh
sostoyaniy (On the study of mechanisms of recovery and experimental
therapy of allergic states). In *Voprosy immunopatologii* (Problems of immunopathology), 21–26. Moscow.

Cherry, C. P.; Eisenstein, R.; and Glucksmanu, A. 1967. Epithelial cords
and tubules of the rat thymus: Effects of age, sex, castration, thyroid and
other hormones on their incidence and secretory activity. *Brit. J. Exp.
Path.* 48:90–106.

Chtetsov, V. P. 1969. *Matematicheskiye metody v biologii* (Mathematical
methods in biology). Moscow.

Chubukhchiyev, V. Kh.; Polyak, A. I.; and Belovolova, R. A. 1976. K soz-
daniyu informatsionnoy modeli bioregulirovaniya immunogo otveta v
organizme (The development of an information model of bioregulation
of the immune response in the organism). In *Mekhanizmy povrezhdeniya, rezistentnosti, adaptatsii i kompensatsii. Tez. dokl.* (Mechanisms of
injury, resistance, adaptation, and compensation. Proceedings), 2:611–
12. Tashkent.

Claman, H. N. 1975. How corticosteroids work. *J. Allergy Clin. Immunol.*
55:145–51.

Cohen, E. P.; Fischbach, M.; and Claman, H. N. 1970. Hydrocortisone resistance of graft host activity in mouse thymus, spleen and bone marrow.
J. Immunol. 105:1146–50.

Cohen, J. J. 1971. The effects of hydrocortisone on the immune response.
Ann. Allergy 29:358–61.

Cohen, P., and Gershon, R. K. 1975. The role of cortisone-sensitive thymo-
cites in DNA synthetic responses to antigen. *Ann. N.Y. Acad. Sci.*
249:451–61.

Corson, S. A. 1957. Review of F. R. Borodulin, S. P. Botkin, and the neurogenic theory of medicine. *Science* 125(3237):75–77.

Corson, S. A., and Corson, E. O'L. 1975. Cerebrovisceral physiology and

pathophysiology and psychosomatic medicine. *Totus Homo* 6(1–3):85–123.

Cox, D. R., and Lewis, P. A. 1969. *Statisticheskiy analiz posledovatel-'nosti sobytiy* (Statistical analysis of sequential events). Moscow.

Craddock et al. 1967a. Cited in Savchuk (1955).

Craddock, C. S.; Winnelstein, A.; Matsuyki, Y.; and Lawrence, J. S. 1967b. The immune response to foreign red blood cells and the participation of short-lived lymphocytes. *J. Exp. Med.* 125:1149–72.

Criep, L. H.; Mayer, L. D.; Menchaca, O. E. L. 1951. The effect of adrenalectomy on experimental hypersensitiveness. *J. Allergy Clin. Immunol.* 22:314–29.

Cross, B. A., and Green, G. D. 1959. Activity of single neurones in the hypothalamus: Effects of osmotic and other stimuli. *J. Physiol.* 148:554–69.

Cross, B. A., and Kitay, G. J. 1967. Unit activity in diencephalic islands. *Exp. Neurol.* 19:316–60.

Cross, B. A., and Silver, I. A. 1963. Unit activity in the hypothalamus and the sympathetic response to hypoxia and hypercapnea. *Exp. Neurol.* 7:375–93.

————. 1965. Effect of luteal hormone on the behaviour of hypothalamic neurones in pseudopregnant rats. *J. Endocrinol.* 31:251–63.

Dafny, N., and Feldman, S. 1970. Unit responses and convergence of sensory stimuli in the hypothalamus. *Brain Res.* 17:243–57.

Danilova, O. A.; Bertash, V. I.; and Ryzhenkov, V. Ye. 1972. Vliyaniye etimizola, AKTG i gidrokortizona na gipotalamo-giofizarnuyu neyrosekretornuyu sistemu morskikh svinok (The influence of ethymisol, adrenocorticotrophic hormone, and hydrocortisone on the hypothalamohypophyseal neurosecretory system in guinea pigs). *Probl. Endokrin.* 18(5):76–80.

Darrach, M. 1959. Effect of steroids on antibody production *in vivo*. In *Mechanisms of hypersensitivity*, 599–612. Boston-Toronto-London.

Darzynkiewicz, Z., and Pienkowski, M. 1969. Effect of prednisolone on RNA synthesis in human lymphocytes stimulated by PHA. *Exp. Cell. Res.* 54:289–92.

Daughaday, W. H. 1959. Steroid protein interactions. *Physiol. Rev.* 39:885–902.

Delespesse, G.; Pochet, R.; Gossart, B.; and Vanderbroeck, J. 1980. Correlation between the number of β-adrenergic receptors and c-AMP synthesis induced by isoproterenol in thymocytes and spleen cells. In *Proceedings of the Fourth International Congress of Immunology*, Paris.

Denisenko, P. P., and Cherednichenko, R. P. 1972. M-kholinreaktivnyye biokhimicheskiye sistemy i obrazovaniye syvorotochnykh antitel (M-cho-

line reactive biochemical systems and the formation of serum antibodies). *Byull, Eksp. Biol. I Med.* 73(4):65–68.

Denisenko, Ye. N. 1970. Vliyaniye nekotorykh otdelov nervnoy sistemy na soderzhaniye 17-oksikortikosteroidov v dinamike generalizovannogo fenomena Shvartsmana (The influence of some sections of the nervous system on the content of 17-hydroxycorticosteroids in the dynamics of the Shwartzman generalized phenomenon). In *Mekhanizmy nekotorykh patologicheskikh protsessov* (The mechanisms of certain pathologic processes), 3:210–15. Rostov-on-Don.

Dertouzos, M. 1967. *Porogovaya logika* (Threshold logic). Moscow.

Devoyno, L. V. 1975. Znachimost' mezo-gipotalamicheskoy serotoninergicheskoy sistemy dlya konstruktsii immunogo otveta (The significance of the mesohypothalamic serotoninergic system for the construction of immune responses). In *Neyrogumoral'naya i farmakologicheskaya korrektsiya immunologicheskikh reaktsiy v eksperimente i klinike.* Tez. dokl. (Neurohumoral and pharmacological correction of immune reactions under experimental and clinical conditions. Proceedings), 18–19. Leningrad.

Devoyno, L. V., and Al'perina, Ye. L. 1982. Vzaimodeystviye dofaminergicheskoy i serotoninergicheskoy sistemy v regulyatsii immunnogo otveta (The interaction of the dopaminergic and serotoninergic systems in the regulation of the immune response). In *Materialy dokladov III vsesoyuznogo simpoziuma "Regulyatsiya immunnogo gomeostaza"* (Proceedings of the third all-union symposium "The regulation of immune homeostasis"), 48–50. Leningrad.

Dews, P. B., and Code, C. F. 1953. Anaphylactic reactions and concentrations of antibody in rats and rabbits: Effect of adrenalectomy and of administration of cortisone. *J. Immunol.* 70:199–206.

Dolin, A. O. 1951. Patologicheskoye i zashchitno-okhranitel'noye v uslovnykh i bezuslovnykh reaktsiyakh (Pathological and defense-protective aspects in conditioned and unconditioned reactions). *Zh. Vyssh. Nervn. Deyat. Im. I. P. Pavlova* 1(6):934–43.

Dolin, A. O., and Krylov, V. N. 1952. Eksperimental'noye izucheniye roli kory golovnogo mozga v immunnykh reaktsiyakh organizma (Experimental study of the role of the cerebral cortex in immune reactions of the organism). *Zh. Vyssh. Nervn. Deyat. Im. I. P. Pavlova* 2(4):547–60.

Dolin, A. O.; Krylov, V. N.; and Luk'yanenko, V. I. 1963. Uslovnyy immunobiologicheskiy refleks (The conditioned immunobiological reflex). In *Tez. dokladov 19-go soveshch. po probl. vysshey nervnoy deyatel'nosti* (Proceedings of the nineteenth conference on problems of higher nervous activity), 93–94. Leningrad.

Dougherty, T. F. 1953. Some observations on mechanisms of corticosteroid

acta on inflammation and immunologic processes. *Ann. N. Y. Acad. Sci.* 56:748–56.

Dougherty, T. F., and Schneebeli, G. L. 1950. Role of cortisone in regulation of inflammation. *Proc. Soc. Exp. Biol. Med.* 75:854–59.

———. 1955. The use of steroids as anti-inflammatory agents. *Ann. N. Y. Acad. Sci.* 61:328–48.

Dougherty, T. F., and White, A. 1947. An evaluation of alterations produced in lymphoid tissue by pituitary-adrenal corticoid secretions. *J. Lab. Clin. Med.* 32:584–605.

Dougherty, T. F.; Berliner, M. L.; and Berliner, D. L. 1960. Hormonal influence on lymphocyte differentiation from RES cells. *Ann. N. Y. Acad. Sci.* 88:78–82.

Dougherty, T. F.; Berliner, M. L.; Schneebeli, G. L.; and Berliner, D. L. 1964. Hormonal control of lymphatic structure and function. *Ann. N. Y. Acad. Sci.* 113:825–43.

Ducor, P., and Dietrich, F. M. 1968. Characteristic features of immunosuppression by steroid and cytotoxic drugs. *Intern. Arch. Allergy Appl. Immunol.* 34:32–48.

Dugueskoy, R. J.; Mariani, T.; and Good, R. A. 1969. Cited in Kalden et al. (1970).

Dugueskoy, R. J.; Kalpaktsoglon, P. K.; and Good, R. A. 1970. Immunological studies of the Snell-Bagg pituitary dwarf mouse. *Proc. Soc. Exp. Biol. Med.* 133:201–6.

Dunn, J. D.; Schindler, W. J.; Hutchins, M. D.; Scheving, L. E.; and Turpen, C. 1973–74. Daily variation in rat growth hormone concentration and the effect of stress on periodicity. *Neuroendocrinology* 13:69–78.

D'yachenko, S. S. 1966. Vliyaniye adrenokortikotropnogo gormona, kortizona i prednizolona na obrazovaniye antitel (The influence of adrenocorticotrophic hormone, cortisone, and prednisolone on the formation of antibodies). In *Voprosy immunologii* (Problems of immunology), 2:51–53. Kiev.

Eastman, C. J.; Ekins, R. P.; Leith, I. M.; and Williams, E. S. 1974. Thyroid hormone response to prolonged cold exposure in man. *J. Physiol.* 241:175–81.

Eisenstein, A. 1973. Effects of adrenal cortical hormones on carbohydrate, protein, and fat metabolism. *Amer. J. Clin. Nutr.* 26:113–20.

Eives, M. W.; Gongh, J.; and Israels, M. C. G. 1964. The place of the lymphocyte in the reticulo-endothelial system: A study of the *in vitro* effect of prednisolone on lymphocytes. *Acta Haematol.* 32:100–107.

Enenkel, H. J., and Pedal, H. W. 1955. Vegetatives Nervensystem und Immunität. 1. Über den Einfluss des vegetativen Nervensystems auf die Bildung des Diphtherie-Antitoxins beim Kaninchen. *Arch. Exp. Path. Pharmakol.* 226:69–77.

Engelhardt, G., and Lendle, L. 1959. Experimentelle Untersuchungen zur Frage anaphylaktischer Reaktionen in Abhängigkeit vom Nervensystem. *Klin. Wschr.* 37:867–73.

Ernstrom, U., and Larson, B. 1966. Thymic and thoracic duct contribution to blood lymphocytes in normal and thyroxin treated guinea-pigs. *Acta Physiol. Scand.* 66:189–95.

Eskin, I. A. 1968. *Osnovy fiziologii endokrinnykh zhelez* (Principles of the physiology of the endocrine glands). Moscow.

Esteban, J. N. 1968. The differential effect of hydrocortisone on the short-lived small lymphocyte. *Anat. Rec.* 162:349–58.

Fabris, N. 1973. Immunodepression in thyroid-deprived animals. *Clin. Exp. Immunol.* 15:601–11.

Fabris, N., and Corda. 1973. Cited in: Fabris (1973).

Fabris, N.; Pierpaoli, W.; and Sorkin, E. 1970. Hormones and the immune response. In *Symposium on "Developmental aspects of antibody formation and structure,"* 79–95. Prague.

Fagraens, A. 1952. Role of ACTH and cortisone in resistance and immunity. *Acta Path. Microbiol. Scand. Suppl.* 93:20–28.

Fanci, A. S. 1975. Mechanisms of corticosteroid action on lymphocyte subpopulations. 1. Redistribution of circulating T and B lymphocytes to the bone marrow. *Immunology* 28:669–80.

Fedorov, Yu. V. 1965. O vliyanii nekotorykh farmakologicheskikh preparatov na vyrabotku spetsificheskikh antitel pri kleshchevom entsefalite v eksperimente (On the influence of some drugs on the production of specific antibodies in experimental tick-borne encephalitis). In *Nauchnyye osnovy proizvodstva vaktsin i syvorotok* (Scientific principles of the production of vaccines and serums), 253–60. Moscow.

Fedoseyev, G. V.; Varnacheva, T. F.; Zhikharev, S. S.; Kotenko, T. V.; Lavrova, O. V.; Malovichko, N. A.; and Mineyev, V. N. 1982. Izmeneniye adrenoreaktivnosti leykotsitov bol'nykh KhNZL v protsesse immunologicheskoy stimulyatsii (Changes in the adrenoreactivity of leukocytes in patients in the process of immune stimulation). In *Materialy dokladov III vsesoyuznogo simpoziuma "Regulyatsiya immunnogo gomeostaza"* (Proceedings of the third all-union symposium "The regulation of immune homeostasis"), 240–42. Leningrad.

Fedotov, V. P., and Sokolov, A. Ya. 1970. Radioimmunologicheskiy metod opredeleniya belkovykh i polipeptidnykh gormonov v plazme krovi (obzor literatury) (The radioimmunologic method of determining protein and polypeptide hormones in the blood plasma. A literature survey). *Probl. Endokrinol.* 16(4):103–10.

Feldman, S., and Dafny, N. 1970. Effects of cortisol on unit activity in the hypothalamus of the rat. *Exp. Neurol.* 27:375–87.

Fernandes, G.; Yunis, E.; Nelson, W.; and Halberg, F. 1974. Differences in

immune response of mice to sheep red blood cells as a function of circadian phase. In *Chronobiology*, 329–35. Stuttgart-Tokyo.

Fialkow, P.; Gillchrist, C.; and Allison, L. 1973. Autoimmunity in chronic graft-versus-host disease. *Clin. Exp. Immunol.* 13:479–86.

Fifkova, E., and Marschal, D. 1962. Sterotaksicheskiy atlas koshki, krolika i krysy (Sterotaxic atlas of the cat, the rabbit, and the rat). In *Elektrofiziologicheskiye metody issledovaniya* (Electrophysiological methods of investigation), ed. Ya Buresh, M. Petran', and I. Zakhar, 384–426. Moscow.

Filimonov, V. G. 1962. Izmeneniye elektrofiziologicheskikh pokazateley kory golovnogo mozga, gipotalamusa i bluzhdayushchego nerva pod vliyaniyem sensibilizatsii organizma (The change of electrophysiological indexes of the cerebral cortex, the hypothalamus, and the vagus nerve under the influence of sensitization of the organism). *Patol. Fiziol. I Eksperim. Terap.* 6(5):45–51.

Filipp, G. 1971. Rol'nervnoy sistemy v allergicheskikh reaktsiyakh (The role of the nervous system in allergic reactions). In *Problemy immunologicheskoy reaktivnosti i allergii* (Problems of immune reactivity and allergy), 166–77. Moscow.

———. 1973. Mechanism of suppressing anaphylaxis through electrolytic lesion of the tuberal region of the hypothalamus. *Ann. Allergy* 31(6):272–78.

Filipp, G., and Mess, B. 1969a. Role of the adrenocortical system in suppressing anaphylaxis after hypothalamic lesion. *Ann. Allergy* 27:607–10.

———. 1969b. Role of the thyroid hormone system in suppressing of anaphylaxis due to electrolytic lesion of the tuberal region of the hypothalamus. *Ann. Allergy*, 27:500–505.

Filipp, G., and Szentiványi, A. 1956. Die Wirkung von Hypothalamusläsionen auf den anaphylaktischen Schock des Meerschweinchens. In *Allergie und Asthmaforschung*, 1:23–28. Dresden.

———. 1958. Anaphylaxis and the nervous system. 3. *Ann. Allergy* 16:306–11.

Filipp, G.; Szentiványi, A.; and Mess, B. 1952. Anaphylaxis and the nervous system. 1. *Acta Med. Acad. Sci.* 3(2):163–73.

Findlay, A. L. R., and Hayward, J. N. 1969. Spontaneous activity of single neurones in the hypothalamus of rabbits during sleep and waking. *J. Physiol.* 201:237–58.

Firsova, P. P. 1953. Fagotsitoz i medikamentnyy son (Phagocytosis and drug-induced sleep). *Vrachebnoye Delo* 2:177–78.

Fischel, E. E. 1953. Cited in Rose (1959).

Fischel, E. E.; Vanghan, J. H.; and Photopoulos, C. 1952. Inhibition of

rapid production of antibody by cortisone: Study of secondary response. In *Proceedings Soc. Exp. Biol. Med.* 81:344–48.

Floerscheim, G. L. 1970. A comparative study of the effects of antitumour and immunosuppressive drugs on antibody forming and erythropoietic cells. *Clin. Exp. Immunol.* 6:861–70.

Franchimont, P.; Legros, J. J.; and Schaub, J. C. 1970. Exploration de l'axe hypothalamo-hypophyso-somatotrope. *Rev. Franc. Endocrinol. Clin. Nutr. Metabol.* 11:105–19.

Freedman, D. X., and Fenichel, G. 1958. Effect of midbrain lesion on experimental allergy. *Arch. Neurol. Psychiat.* 79:164–69.

Fridenshteyn, A. Ya., and Chertkov, I. L. 1969. *Kletochnyye osnovy immuniteta* (Cellular principles of immunity). Moscow.

Frolov, Ye. P. 1974. *Neuro-gumoral'nyye mekhanizmy regulyatsii immunologicheskikh protsessov* (Neurohumoral mechanisms of regulation of immune processes). Moscow.

Frolov, Ye. P.; Kozlov, V. K.; Giber, L. M.; and Shatilova, N. V. 1972. Simpaticheskaya nervnaya sistema kak efferentnoye zveno regulyatsii immunologicheskoy reaktivnosti (The sympathetic nervous system as the efferent component in the regulation of immune reactivity). In *Problemy sovremennoy immunobiologii* (Problems of modern immunobiology), 260–62. Moscow.

Frolov, Ye. P.; Kozlov, V. K.; and Rodionov, I. M. 1972. Novyye dannyye o roli simpaticheskoy nervnoy sistemy v regulyatsii obrazovaniya antitel i v razvitii anafilakticheskogo shoka (New data on the role of the sympathetic nervous system in the regulation of antibody formation and in the development of anaphylactic shock). *Patol. Fiziol.* 4:79–82.

Frolov, Ye. P.; Undritsov, M. I.; and Shatilova, N. V. 1972. Funktsional'nyye sdvigi i formirovaniye spetsificheskoy reaktivnosti pri sensibilizatsii krolikov tsitoplazmaticheskimi antigenami A-streptokokka (Functional changes and development of specific reactivity upon sensitization of rabbits with cytoplasmic antigens of A-streptococcus). *Patol. Fiziol.* 5:38–43.

Frolov, Ye. P.; Serebryakov, N. G.; Vasina, I. G.; and Shatilova, N. V. 1973. Napravlennyye izmeneniya immunologicheskoy reaktivnosti s pomoshch'yu vmeshatel'stva v neyrogumoral'nyye mekhanizmy (Directed changes in immune reactivity by means of intervention in neurohumoral mechanisms). In *Immunodepressiya pri transplantatsii organov* (Immune depression in organ transplantation), 45–56. Moscow.

Gabourel, J. D., and Comstock, J. P. 1964. Effect of hydrocortisone on amino acid incorporation by microsomes isolated from mouse lymphoma ML-388 cells and rat thymus. *Biochem. Pharmacol.* 13:1369–76.

Gamaleya, N. F. 1928. *Osnovy immunologii* (Principles of immunology). Moscow-Leningrad.

Ganenko, D. M. 1969. *Problemy differentsial'noy psikhofiziologii* (Problems of differential psychophysiology), vol. 6. Moscow.

Garkavi, L. Kh. 1962. Vliyaniye razdrazheniy gipotalamusa na rost perevivayemykh sarkom (The influence of stimulation of the hypothalamus on the growth of transplanted sarcomas. Dissertation). Rostov-on-Don.

Gaumer, H. R.; Salvaggio, J. E.; Weston, W. L.; and Claman, H. N. 1974. Cortisol inhibition of immunologic activity in guinea pig alveolar cells. *Intern. Arch. Allergy Appl. Immunol.* 47:797–809.

Gavrilova, L. N. 1954. Dannyye k voprosu o razdel'nosti gormonov zadney doli gipofiza (Data on the question of the distinctiveness of the hormones of the posterior lobe of the hypophysis). *Fiziol. Zhurn. SSSR* 40(1):60–64.

Gellhorn, E. 1967. *Autonomic imbalance and the hypothalamus.* Minneapolis: University of Minnesota Press.

Germanov, N. I. 1953. Produktsiya antitel v usloviyakh tormozheniya nervnoy sistemy (The production of antibodies under conditions of inhibition of the nervous system). *Zhurn. Mikrobiol., Epidemiol., Immunobiol.* 24(12):33–41.

Gerstein, G. L., and Kiang, N. Y. S. 1960. An approach to the quantitative analysis of electrophysiological data from single neurons. *Biophys. J.* 1:215–34.

Gisler, R. H., and Schenkel-Hullinger, L. 1971. Hormonal regulation of the immune response. 2. Influence of pituitary and adrenal activity on immune responsiveness *in vitro. Cell. Immunol.* 2:646:51.

Gisler, R. H.; Bussard, A. E.; Mazie, J. C.; and Hess, R. 1971. Hormonal regulation of the immune response. 1. Induction of an immune response *in vitro* with lymphoid cells from mice exposed to acute systemic stress. *Cell. Immunol.* 2:634–45.

Glazyrina, P. V. 1958. K voprosu o korkovoy regulyatsii serdechnoy deyatel'nosti pri sensibilizatsii belkovym antigenom (On the question of the cortical regulation of cardiac activity upon sensitization with protein antigen. Dissertation). Chelyabinsk.

Glezer, V. D.; Troshikhina, Yu. G.; and Dashin, I. I. 1966. O kodirovanii yarkosti neyronami zritel'noy kory koshki (On the coding of brightness by neurons of the visual cortex of the cat). In *DAN SSSR* (Proceedings of the Academy of Sciences of the USSR), 170(6):1443–46.

Glezer, V. D.; Dudkin, K. N.; Ivanov, V. A.; and Kul'kov, A. P. 1968. O kodirovanii signalov v impul'snykh posledovatel'nostyakh (Signal coding in pulse sequences). In *Statisticheskaya elektrofiziologiya* (Statistical electrophysiology), 1:141–55. Vilnius.

Glick, B., and Schwarz, M. R. 1975. Thymidine and testosterone incorporation by bursal and thymic lymphocytes. *Immunol. Commun.* 4(2):123–37.

Glick, S. M.; Roth, J.: Jalow, R. S.; and Berson, S. A. 1965. The regulation of growth hormone secretion. *Rec. Progr. Horm. Res.* 21:241–70.

Glotova, Ye. V.; Vakhmistrova, Ye. V.; and Ignatovich, Z. A. 1931. Vliyaniye nekotorykh fizicheskikh faktorov na agglyutininy (The influence of certain physical factors on agglutinins). *Zhurn. Mikrobiol., Epidemiol., Immunobiol.* 8(2):132–35.

Gogolitsin, Yu. L. 1975. Analiz protsessov kodirovaniya verbal'nykh signalov golovnym mozgom cheloveka (Analysis of processes of the coding of verbal signals by the human brain. Dissertation). Leningrad.

Gol'dshteyn, M. M. 1971. K voprosu o vozmozhnoy roli struktur zadnego gipotalamusa v mekhanizme antiteloobrazovaniya (On the question of a possible role of structures of the posterior hypothalamus in the mechanism of antibody formation). In *Problemy allergii v klinike i eksperimente*. Tez. dokladov (Problems of allergy under clinical and experimental conditions. Proceedings), 33–34. Moscow.

Golikov, N. V. 1950. Fiziologicheskaya labil'nost' i yeye izmeneniya pri osnovnykh nervnykh protsessakh (Physiological lability and its changes during basic neural processes). Leningrad.

———. 1965. *Dostizheniya sovremennoy fiziologii nervnoy i myshechnoy sistemy* (Advances in the modern physiology of the nervous and muscular system). Moscow-Leningrad.

Golodets, G. G., and Puchkov, N. V. 1948. O vliyanii mediatorov na fagotsitarnuyu deyatel'nost' leykotsitov (On the influence of mediators on the phagocytic activity of leukocytes). *Fiziol. Zhurn. SSSR* 34(1):135–42.

Golovkova, I. N. 1947. O vliyanii bolevogo i uslovnoreflektornogo razdrazheniya na fagotsitarnuyu sposobnost' leykotsitov v organizme (The influence of painful and conditioned reflex stimulation on the phagocytic capacity of leukocytes in the organism). *Byull. Eksper. Biol. I Med.* 24(1):268–70.

Golubeva, N. N., and Marat, B. A. 1972. Reaktivnyye svoystva kul'tur limfotsitov perifericheskoy krovikrolikovs povrezhdeniyem gipotalamicheskikh struktur (Reactive properties of cultures of lymphocytes of the peripheral blood in rabbits with damaged hypothalamic structures). *Byull. Eksp. Biol. I Med.* 74(11):85–87.

Golubeva, N. N.; Korneva, Ye. A.; Shul'gina, N. S.; Savchuk, L. N.; Pikhtar', V. I.; and Marat, B. A. 1971. Rol'gumoral'nogo i kletochnogo faktorov immunogeneza v protsesses prizhivleniya transplantata rogovoy obolochki (The role of humoral and cellular factors in the process of acceptance of corneal transplants). In *Osobennosti proyavleniy tkanevoy*

nesovmestimosti pri transplantatsii organov. Mater. simpoz. (Character-istics of the manifestation of tissue incompatibility in organ transplanta-tion. Proceedings of symposium), 98–100. Moscow.

Golubeva, N. N.; Vardanyan, I. K.; and Golubeva, V. F. 1975. K voprosu vzaimodeystviya neyromediatorov i mediatorov immunnogo otveta i me-todicheskiye podkhody v izuchenii etikh vzaimodeystviy na kletochnom urovne (On the question of interaction of neuromediators and mediators of the immune response and methodical approaches in the study of these interactions at the cellular level). In *Neyrogumoral'naya i farmakologi-cheskaya korrektsiya immunologicheskikh reaktsiy v eksperimente i klin-ike.* Tez. dokladov (Neurohumoral and pharmacologic correction of im-mune reactions under experimental and clinical conditions. Proceedings), 14–45. Leningrad.

Golubeva, N. N.; Vardanyan, I. K.; Seskavina, L. S.; and Sitkovskiy, M. V. 1979. K voprosu o vzaimodeystvii noradrenalina i al'faadrenoblo-katorov s limfoidnymi kletkami (The problem of the interaction of nora-drenaline and alpha-adrenergic blocking agents with lymphoid cells). *Fi-ziol. Zh. SSSR* 65(6):627–33.

Golubeva, N. N.; Gordon, D. S.; Vardanyan, I. K.; Lavrov, V. F.; Marko-syan, K. M.; Gudkova, Yu. V.; and Kononova, T. D. 1982. Dozovaya zavisimost' moduliruyushchego effekta nekotorykh mediatorov i gor-monov na rannikh etapakh aktivatsii limfotsitov (The dose dependence of the modulating effect of certain mediators and hormones at early stages of the activation of the lymphocytes). In *Materialy dokladov III Vsesoyuznogo simpoziuma "Regulyatsiya immunnogo gomeostaza"* (Proceedings of the third all-Union symposium "The regulation of im-mune homeostasis"), 137–38. Leningrad.

Gorbunova, L. V. 1975. Vliyaniye zadnikh yader gipotalamusa na nekotor-yye immunologicheskiye reaktsii povyshennoy chuvstvitel'nosti zamed-lennogo i nemedlennogo tipov (The influence of the posterior nuclei of the hypothalamus on certain immune reactions of raised sensitivity of the delayed and the immediate type. Dissertation). Gor'kii.

Gordiyenko, A. N. 1949. *Nervnaya sistema i immunitet* (The nervous sys-tem and immunity). Krasnodar.

―――. 1954. *Nervnoreflektornyy mekhanizm vyrabotki antitel i regulyat-siya fagotsitoza* (The neuroreflex mechanism of the production of anti-bodies and the regulation of phagocytosis). Moscow.

―――. 1965. *Eksperimental'naya immunopatologiya* (Experimental im-munopathology). Kiev.

Gordiyenko, A. N.; Kiseleva, V. I.; Saakov, B. A.; Bondarev, I. M.; and Zhigalina, L. I. 1958. K mekhanizmu deystviya antigena na retseptory

karotidnogo sinusa pri reflektornoy vyrabotke antitel (On the mechanism of antigen action on the receptors of the carotid sinus in the reflex production of antibodies). In *Nervnaya regulyatsiya immunogeneza* (The nervous regulation of immunogenesis), 129–34. Rostov-on-Don.

Gordon, D. S.; Sergeyeva, V. Ye.; and Golubeva, N. N. 1982. Gistokhimicheskiye kriterii otsenki neyromediatornogo statusa limfoidnykh organov pri antigennom i nespetsificheskom vozdeystviyakh na organizm (Histochemical criteria for determining the neuromediator status of the lymph organs during antigenic and nonspecific actions on the organism). In *Materialy dokladov III Vsesoyuznogo simpoziuma "Regulyatsiya immunnogo gomeostaza"* (Proceedings of the third all-Union symposium "The regulation of immune homeostasis"), 12–13. Leningrad.

Gordon, M. A.; Cohen, J. J.; and Wilson, I. B. 1978. Muscarinic cholinergic receptors in murine lymphocytes: Demonstration by direct binding. In *Proc. Natl. Acad. Sci. U.S.A.*, 75(6):2902–4.

Grachev, G. I., and Stepushkina, T. A. 1968. Statisticheskaya kharakteristika fonovoy aktivnosti efferentnykh neyronov i yeye funktsional'noye znacheniye (Statistical characteristics of the background activity of efferent neurons and its functional significance). In *Statisticheskaya elektrofiziologiya. Mater. simpoz.* (Statistical electrophysiology. Proceedings of symposium), 2:217–24. Vilnius.

Granit, R. 1955. *Receptors and sensory perception*. New Haven: Yale University Press.

———. 1957. *Elektrofiziologicheskoye issledovaniye retseptsiy* (An electrophysiological study of receptors). Moscow.

Grashchenkov, N. I. 1964. *Gipotalamus: yego rol' v fiziologii i patologii* (The hypothalamus: Its role in physiology and pathology). Moscow.

Green, G. D., and Morin, F. 1953. Hypothalamic electrical activity and hypothalamocortical relationships. *Amer. J. Physiol.* 172:175.

Grigor'yev, V. A. 1982. Dinamika urovnya postoyannogo potentsiala gipotalamicheskikh struktur krolikov v protsesse razvitiya immunnykh reaktsiy (The dynamics of the level of the steady-state potential of the hypothalamic structures of rabbits during the development of immune responses. Dissertation). Leningrad.

Gromova, Ye. A.; Tkachenko, K. N.; and Provodina, V. N. 1964. K funktsional'noy kharakteristike gipotalamusa (On the functional characteristics of the hypothalamus). In *Tr. In-ta Norm. i Patol. Fiziol. AMN SSSR* (Proceedings of the Institute of Normal and Pathological Physiology of the Academy of Medical Sciences of the USSR), 7:37–38.

Groot, J. de, and Harris, G. 1950. Hypothalamic control of the anterior pituitary gland and blood lymphocytes. *J. Physiol.* 111:335–46.

Grossman, R. G., and Viernstein, L. J. 1961. Discharge patterns of neurons in cochlear nucleus. *Science* 134:99-101.

Gubler, Ye. V., and Genkin, A. A. 1973. *Primeneniye kriteriyev neparametricheskoy statistiki v medikobiologicheskikh issledovaniyakh* (The application of criteria of nonparametric statistics in medicobiological investigations). Leningrad.

Gurvich, G. A. 1963. Deystviye dezoksikortikosterona i somatotrofnogo gormona na immunyye reaktsii organizma (The effect of desoxycorticosterone and somatotropic hormone on immune reactions of the organism). In *Voprosy infektsionnoy patologii i immunologii* (Problems of infectious pathology and immunology), 3:29-35. Moscow.

Gushchin, G. V. 1975. Immunnoye rozetkoobrazovaniye u lineynykh myshey na fone vvedeniya nekotorykh neyrotropnykh preparatov (Immune rosette formation in inbred mice on the background of administration of some neurotropic preparations). In *Neyrogumoral'naya i farmakologicheskaya korrektsiya immunologicheskikh reaktsiy v eksperimente i klinike. Tez. dokladov* (Proceedings of neurohumoral and pharmacologic correction of immune reactions under experimental and clinical conditions), 16-17. Leningrad.

Gushchin, I. S. 1962. K uchastiyu gipotalamusa v razvitii anafilaktoidnogo shoka u belykh krys (On the participation of the hypothalamus in the development of anaphylactic shock in white rats). In *Voprosy patologicheskoy fiziologii infektsionnogo protsessa* (Problems of the pathophysiology of the infectious process), 149-55. Moscow.

Hadden, J. W.; Hadden, E. M.; and Middleton, E. 1970. lymphocyte blast transformation. 1. Demonstration of adrenergic receptors in human peripheral lymphocytes. *Cell. Immunol.* 1:583-95.

Hagiwara, S. 1954. Analysis of interval fluctuation of the sensory nerve impulse. *J. Physiol. Jap.* 234-40.

Halliday, W. J., and Garvey, J. S. 1964a. Hydrocortisone and the apparent induction period for antibody formation *in vitro*. *Nature* 202:712-13.

_____. 1964b. Some factors affecting the secondary immune response in tissue culture containing hydrocortisone. *J. Immunol.* 93:757-62.

Hammond, C. W., and Novak, M. 1950. Relation of adrenal cortical steroids to antibody release. In *Proc. Soc. Exp. Biol. Med.*, 155-61.

Han, T. 1974a. Immunosuppressive effect of human chorionic gonadotropin on cell-mediated immunity *in vitro* and *in vivo*. *Blood* 44:921.

_____. 1974b. Inhibitory effect of human chorionic gonadotrophin on lymphocyte blastogenic response to mitogen, antigen and allogeneic cells. *Clin. Exp. Immunol.* 18:529-35.

_____. 1975. Human chorionic gonadotropin: Its inhibitory effect on cell-mediated immunity *in vivo* and *in vitro*. *Immunology* 29:509-15.

Hangen, S.; Basse, H. H.; and Flood, P. R. 1969. Phagocytosis in rabbits treated with oxyphenbutazone and cortisone: Studied by gold clearance test and electron microscopy. *J. Reticul. Soc.* 6:184–89.

Hanjan, S. N. S., and Talwar, G. P. 1975. Effect of growth hormone on surface charge and electrophoretic mobility of thymocytes from young and aged rats. *Molec. Cell. Endocrinol.* 3:185–201.

Hansen, H. G. 1957. Über den Wirkungsmechanismus der Nebennierenrindenhormone am lymphatischen System. In *Proc. Sixth Congr. Europ. Soc. Haematol. Kopenhagen*, 2:59.

Haolden, J. W. 1975. Cyclic nucleotides in lymphocyte function. *Ann. N. Y. Acad. Sci.* 256:352–64.

Havlicek, V., and Sklenovsky, A. 1967. Effect of noradrenaline on the unit activity in hypothalamus. *Activ. Nerv. Sup.* (Praha) 9:190–92.

Hayashida, T., and Li, C. H. 1957. The influence of adrenocorticotropic and growth hormones on antibody formation. *J. Exp. Med.* 105:93–98.

Heller, I. 1955. Cortisone and phagocytosis. *Endocrinology* 56:80–85.

Hilgar, A. G. 1968. The thymolitic evaluation of steroids and other compounds. In *Thymolitic and glycogenic endocrine bioassay data*, 2:1–3. Bethesda, Md.: National Institutes of Health.

Hill, C. W.; Greer, W. E.; and Felsenfeld, O. 1967. Psychological stress, early response to foreign protein and blood cortisol in monkeys. *Psychosom. Med.* 29:279–83.

Hirsch, J. G., and Church, A. B. 1961. Adrenal steroids and infection: The effect of cortisone administration on polymorphonuclear leucocyte functions and on serum opsonins and bactericidins. *J. Clin. Invest.* 40:794–98.

Holm, E., and Schaefer, H. 1969. Eine Faktorenanalyse von Schwellen subcorticaler Reizantworten. *Exp. Brain. Res.* 8:79–88.

Holne, R.; Riudani, T. H.; and Heuser, G. 1954. Influence of somatotrophic hormone and hydrocortisone on the production of haematolitic antibodies in the rat. *Amer. J. Physiol.* 177:19–22.

Hsii, E. H., and Cherman, M. 1946. The factor analysis of the electroencephalogram. *J. Psychol.* 21:189–96.

Hunt, C. C., and Kuno, M. 1959. Properties of spinal interneurones. *J. Physiol.* 147:346.

Ingle, D. I. 1954. Permissibility of hormone action. *Acta Endocrinol.* (Kopenhagen), 17:172–86.

Ioffe, V. I., and Rozental', K. M. 1943. Eksperimental'nyye materialy k ob'yasneniyu bol'shey chuvstvitel'nosti metoda dlitel'nogo kholodnogo svyazyvaniya (Experimental material for the explanation of the greater sensitivity of the method of prolonged cold fixation). *Zhurn. Mikrobiol., Epidemiol., Immunobiol.* 14(12):65–68.

Ishidate, J., and Metcalf, D. 1963. The pattern of lymphopoiesis in the mouse thymus after cortisone administration or adrenalectomy. *J. Exp. Biol. Med. Sci., Austral.* 41:637–51.

Ishizuka, M.; Gafni, M.; and Braun, W. 1970. Cyclic AMP effects on antibody formation and their similarities to hormone-mediated events. In *Proc. Soc. Exp. Biol.*, 134:963–67.

Ishizuka, M.; Braun, W.; and Matsumoto, T. 1971. Cyclic AMP and immune responses. *J. Immunol.* 107:1027–35.

Ivanov, V. M. 1963. Vliyaniye adrenalektomii i vvedeniya nekotorykh kortikosteroidov na obrazovaniye antitel (The influence of adrenalectomy and administration of certain corticosteroids on the formation of antibodies). *Vestn. AMN SSSR* 18(11):19–24.

———. 1964. K vliyaniyu kory nadpochechnikov na immunogenez (The influence of the adrenal cortex on immunogenesis). *Patol. Fiziol. I Eksper. Terap.* 8(3):16–19.

Izotov, V. K., and Lazarev, A. F. 1963. K voprosu o vliyanii gormona rosta na effekt immunizatsii virusom kleshchevogo entsefalita (On the influence of growth hormone on the effect of immunization with the virus of tick-borne encephalitis). In *Kleshchevoy entsefalit i virusnyye gemorragicheskiye likhoradki* (Tick-borne encephalitis and viral hemorrhagic fevers), 67–68. Omsk.

Janković, B. D., and Isaković, K. 1973. Neuroendocrine correlates of immune response. 1. Effects of brain lesions on antibody production, Arthus reactivity and delayed hypersensitivity in the rat. *Intern. Arch. Allergy Appl. Immunol.* 45:360–72.

Janković, B. D.; Isaković, K.; and Ivanus, J. 1972. Immune response and lymphatic tissue reaction in brain lesioned rats. In *Fourth international conference on lymphatic tissue and germinal centers in immune reactions.* Abstracts, Dubrovnik, 31.

Jones, W., and Kayc, M. 1973. Investigation of a possible immunosuppressive role for human chorionic gonadotropin in human pregnancy. In *Immunologiya razmnozheniya* (The immunology of reproduction), 665–69. Sofia.

Jong, W., and Moll, J. de. 1965. Differential effects of hypothalamic lesions on pituitary and thyroid. *Acta Endocrinol.* 48:552–55.

Kakhana, M. S. 1961. *Patofiziologiya gipotalamusa* (Pathophysiology of the hypothalamus). Kishinev.

Kalden, Y. R.; Evans, M. M.; and Irvine, W. J. 1970. The effect of hypophysectomy on the immune response. *J. Immunol.* 18:671–80.

Kanarevskaya, A. A. 1937. Rol'nervnoy sistemy v anafilaksii (The role of the nervous system in anaphylaxis). *Arch. Biol. Nauk* 45(7):83–101.

Kanda, R. 1959a. Studies of the regulation centre on promotion of anti-

body. 1. On the migrations of agglutinin-titer on the peripheral blood by the electric stimuli in hypothalamus of rabbit. *Jap. J. Bacteriol.* 14:223–28.

_____. 1959b. Studies of the regulation centre on promotion of antibody. 2. On the migration and relation of normal precipitin antibody and leucocyte in the peripheral blood by electric stimuli in hypothalamus of rabbit. *Jap. J. Bacteriol.* 14(6):542–45.

Karamyan, A. I. 1959. Nekotoryye voprosy fiziologii retikulyarnoy formatsii s tochki zreniya ucheniya ob adaptatsionnotroficheskoy roli nervnoy sistemy (Some questions of the physiology of the reticular formation from the point of view of the theory of the adaptotrophic role of the nervous system). *Fiziol. Zhurn. SSSR* 45(7):778–88.

Karmali, R. A.; Lander, S.; and Horrobin, D. F. 1974. Prolactin and the immune response. *Lancet* 7872:106–7.

Karpov, M. K. 1952. O nervnom mekhanizme i immunitete pri gazovoy gangrene (On the nervous mechanism and immunity in emphysematous gangrene). *Zhurn. Mikrobiol., Epidemiol., Immunobiol.* 23(11):17–25.

Kass, E. 1960. Protective effect of corticosteroids and of components of normal blood against the lethal action of bacterial lipopolysaccharides. In *Reticuloendothelial structure and function*, 355–64. New York.

Katani, M.; Nawa, G.; and Fujii, H. 1974. Inhibition by testosterone of immune reactivity and of lymphoid regeneration in irradiated and marrow reconstituted mice. *Experientia* 30:1343–45.

Kavetsky, R. E.; Turkevich, N. M.; Akimova, R. N.; Khayetsky, I. K.; and Matveichuck, Y. D. 1969. Induced carcinogenesis under various influences on the hypothalamus. *Ann. N.Y. Acad. Sci.* 164(2):517–19.

Kaznacheyev, V. P., and Subbotin, M. Ya. 1971. *Etyudy k teorii obshchey patologii* (Essays on the theory of general pathology). Novosibirsk.

Kebadze, N. N. 1957. Fagotsitarnaya sposobnost' leykotsitov pri eksperimental'nom tireotoksikoze (The phagocytic ability of leukocytes in experimental thyrotoxicosis). In *Tr. In-ta Eksperim. i Klinich. Khirurgii* (Proceedings of the Institute of Experimental and Clinical Surgery), 355–61. Tbilisi.

Kemp, R. G., and Dugueskoy, R. J. 1975. Lymphoid cell adenylate cyclase activity after X-irradiation and cortisone treatment. *J. Immunol.* 144:660–64.

Kemp, R. G.; Huang, J. Ch.; and Dugueskoy, R. J. 1973. Decreased epinephrine response of adenylate cyclase activity of lymphoid cells from immunodeficient pituitary dwarf mice. *J. Immunol.* 111:1855.

Kesztyüs, L. 1967. *Immunität und Nervensystem.* Budapest.

Khay, L. M. 1956. K izucheniyu nervnoy regulyatsii infektsionnogo

protsessa (The study of neural regulation of the infectious process). In *Osnovy immuniteta* (Principles of immunity), 213–23. Moscow.

Khay, L. M., and Korneva, E. A. 1959. Ob izmenenii serdechnoy deyatel-'nosti u krolikov s yavleniyami autosensibilizatsii (The change in cardiac activity in rabbits with phenomena of autosensitization). In *Tez. dokladov k konf., posvyashch. kompleksnomu izucheniyu problem infektsionnoy patologii* (Proceedings of the conference devoted to the comprehensive study of problems of infectious pathology), 25. Leningrad.

————. 1961. Eksperimental'nyye issledovaniya roli simpato-adrenalovoy sistemy v immunologicheskikh protsessakh. Soobshch. 2. O vliyanii udaleniya mozgovogo sloya nadpochechnikov i vvedeniya aminazina na immunologicheskiye protsessy (Experimental investigations of the role of the sympathoadrenal system in immune processes. Rep. 2. The influence of removal of the adrenal medulla and chlorpromazine administration on immune processes). In *Yezhegodnik IEM za 1960 g.* (Yearbook of the Institute of Experimental Medicine for 1960), 307–13. Leningrad.

Khay, L. M.; Kovalenkova, M. V.; Korneva, E. A.; and Seranova, A. Ye. 1964. Dal'neysheye izucheniye roli gipotalamicheskoy oblasti v regulyatsii protsessa immunogeneza (Further study of the role of the hypothalamic area in the regulation of the process of immunogenesis). *Zhurn. Mikrobiol., Epidemiol., Immunobiol.* 35(10):7–12.

Khlebutina, T. A. 1957. Vliyaniye razdrazheniy podbugornoy oblasti mozga na reaktsii immuniteta (The influence of stimulations of the hypothalamic area of the brain on reactions of immunity. Dissertation). Rostov State University.

————. 1967. Funktsional'noye sostoyaniye i nekotoryye aspekty regulyatsii gipotalamo-gipofizarno-nadpochechnikovoy sistemy v dinamike eksperimental'nogo allergicheskogo entsefalomiyelita (The functional state and some aspects of regulation of the hypothalamohypophyseal-adrenal system in the dynamics of experimental allergic encephalomyelitis. Dissertation). Rostov-on-Don.

Khoruzhaya, T. A., and Vilkov, G. A. 1970. K voprosu ob utilizatsii kortikosteroidnykh gormonov pri eksperimental'nom allergicheskom entsefalomiyelite (On the utilization of corticosteroid hormones in experimental allergic encephalomyelitis). In *Mekhanizmy nekotorykh patologicheskikh protsessov* (Mechanisms of certain pathological processes), 3:197–205. Rostov-on-Don.

Khozak, L. Ye. 1953. Vliyaniye eksperimental'noy sensibilizatsii na rabotu vysshikh otdelov tsentral'noy nervnoy sistemy, v osobennosti kory bol'shikh polushariy golovnogo mozga zhivotnykh (morskiye svinki) (The influence of experimental sensitization on the function of the higher parts

of the central nervous system, especially the cerebral cortex of animals [guinea pigs]). *Zh. Vyssh. Nervn. Deyat. Im. I. P. Pavlova* 3(1):144–55.

Kibyakov, A. V. 1950. *O prirode regulyatornogo vliyaniya simpaticheskoy nervnoy sistemy* (On the nature of the regulatory influence of the sympathetic nervous system). Kazan'.

Kinnaert, P.; Penneman, R.; and Mahieu, A. 1972. Effect of a single large dose of hydrocortisone on phagocytic activity. *Prelim. Rept. Bull. Soc. Int. Chir.* 31:481–86.

Kiseleva, V. I. 1957. Izmeneniye reaktivnosti podkorkovykh obrazovaniy pri sensibilizatsii i anafilakticheskom shoke (The change of reactivity of subcortical formations in sensitization and anaphylactic shock). In *Tr. otchetnoy nauchnoy konf. Rostovskogo Med. In-ta* (Proceedings of the scientific review conference of the Rostov Medical Institute), 45–46.

———. 1960. Elektrofiziologicheskiye izmeneniya v tsentral'noy nervnoy sisteme pri anafilaksii (Electrophysiological changes in the central nervous system in anaphylaxis). In *Problemy kompensatsii, eksperimental'noy terapii i luchevoy bolezni* (Problems of compensation, experimental therapy, and radiation sickness), 107–9. Moscow.

———. 1963a. Elektrofiziologicheskiye issledovaniya nervnykh provodnikov pri anafilakticheskom shoke (Electrophysiological investigations of neural conductors in anaphylactic shock). In *Voprosy immunopatologii* (Problems of immunopathology), 170–72. Moscow.

———. 1963b. Elektrofiziologicheskiye izmeneniya v razlichnykh otdelakh nervnoy sistemy pri anafilaksii (Electrophysiologic changes in various parts of the nervous system in anaphylaxis). In *Elektrofiziologiya nervnoy sistemy* (Electrophysiology of the nervous system), 188–89. Rostov-on-Don.

Kishkovskaya, O. V. 1972a. K gistokhimicheskoy kharakteristike pervichnogo immunologicheskogo otveta (On the histochemical characteristics of the primary immune response). In *Mekhanizmy nekotorykh patologicheskikh protsessov* (Mechanisms of certain pathological processes), 4(2):35–41. Rostov-on-Don.

———. 1972b. Kolichestvennoye izucheniye antiteloobrazuyushchikh kletok limfoidnoy tkani krys v dinamike pervichnogo immunologicheskogo otveta (Quantitative study of antibody-forming cells of the lymphoid tissue of rats in the dynamics of primary immune response). In *Mekhanizmy nekotorykh patologicheskikh protsessov* (Mechanisms of certain pathological processes), 4(2):41–46. Rostov-on-Don.

———. 1974. K gistokhimicheskoy i elektronnomikroskopicheskoy kharakteristike limfoidnoy tkani v protsesse immunogeneza na fone razrusheniya yader zadnego gipotalamusa (On the histochemical and electron-

microscopic characteristics of the lymphoid tissue in the process of immunogenesis on the background of destruction of the nuclei of the posterior hypothalamus). In *Mekhanizmy nekotorykh patologicheskikh protsessov* (Mechanisms of certain pathological processes), 5:167–78. Rostov-on-Don.

Kishkovskaya, O. V.; Zufarov, K. A.; Saakov, B. A.; and Polyak, A. I. 1975. K morfologicheskoy i submikroskopicheskoy kharakteristike pervichnogo immunologicheskogo otveta na fone povrezhdeniya struktur zadnego gipotalamusa (On the morphological and submicroscopic characteristics of primary immune response on the background of damage to structures of the posterior hypothalamus). *Byull. Eksper. Biol. I Med.* 79(1):78–83.

Klegg, P., and Klegg, A. 1971. *Gormony, kletki, organizm* (Hormones, cells, the organism). Moscow.

Klimenko, V. M. 1971. K voprosu ob analize dlitel'notekushchikh nervnykh protsessov v gipotalamuse (On the question of the analysis of prolonged nervous processes in the hypothalamus). In *Tez. dokladov III Vsesoyuznoy konferentsii po fiziologii vegetativnoy nervnoy sistemy* (Proceedings of the third all-Union conference on the physiology of the involuntary nervous system), 105. Yerevan.

————. 1981. Izucheniye vzaimozavisimosti izmeneniy funktsional'nogo sostoyaniya kory bol'shikh polushariy i podkorkovykh struktur v protsesse gomeostaticheskoy deyatel'nosti (A study of the interdependence of the changes in the functional state of the cerebral cortex and the subcortical structures during homeostatic activity). In *Materialy XI Vsesoyuznoy konferentsii po fiziologii i patologii kortiko-vistseral'nykh vzaimootnosheniy* (Proceedings of the eleventh all-Union conference on the physiology and pathology of corticovisceral interrelations), 46–47. Leningrad.

Klimenko, V. M., and Kaplunovskiy, A. S. 1972. Statisticheskoye issledovaniye impul'snoy aktivnosti struktur zadnego gipotalamusa (Statistical investigation of the impulse activity of structures of the posterior hypothalamus). *Fiziol. Zhurn. SSSR* 58(10):1484–93.

Klimenko, V. M.; Kaplunovskiy, A. S.; and Neroslavskiy, I. A. 1972. Avtomaticheskaya klassifikatsiya mnogoparametricheskikh eksperimental'nykh dannykh (Automatic classification of multiparametric experimental data). *Fiziol. Zhurn. SSSR* 58(4):599–602.

Knigge, K. M., and Skott, D. E. 1970. Structure and function of the median eminence. *Amer. J. Anat.* 129:223–28.

Kogan, A. B. 1958. Ob elektrofiziologicheskikh pokazatelyakh vozbuzhdeniya i tormozheniya v kore golovnogo mozga (On electrophysiological indicators of stimulation and inhibition in the cerebral cortex). *Fiziol. Zhurn. SSSR* 44(9):810–19.

_____. 1964. O proyavleniyakh ekologicheskikh osobennostey analizator-noy deyatel'nosti mozga krys i golubey (On the manifestations of ecological features of the analyzer activity of the brain of rats and pigeons). *Fiziol. Zhurn. SSSR* 50(8):934–41.

_____. 1969. *Elektrofiziologiya* (Electrophysiology). Moscow.

Komissarenko, V. P., and Reznikov, A. G. 1972. *Ingibitory funktsii kory nadpochechnikovykh zhelez* (Inhibitors of the function of the adrenal cortex). Kiev.

Konar, D. B., and Manchanda, S. K. 1970. Role of hypothalamus in the activity of reticuloendothelial system. *Indian J. Physiol. Pharmacol.* 14:23–31.

_____. 1972. Hypothalamic influence on the immune response of rats to sheep red blood cells. *Indian J. Physiol. Pharmacol.* 16:277–81.

Konovalov, G. V.; Korneva, Ye. A.; and Khay, L. M. 1971. Vliyaniye razrusheniya zadnego polya gipotalamusa na razvitiye eksperimental'nogo allergicheskogo polinevrita (The influence of the destruction of the posterior area of the hypothalamus on the development of experimental allergic polyneuritis). *Vestn. AMN SSSR* 26(1):60–65.

Kopytovskaya, L. P. 1959. O chuvstvitel'nosti belykh myshey, lishennykh nadpochechnikov, k nekotorym bakteriynym yadam i produktam obmena mikrobov (On the sensitivity of adrenalectomized white mice to certain bacterial poisons and products of microbial metabolism). In *Sovremennye problemy immunologii* (Current problems of immunology), 98–105. Leningrad.

_____. 1970. Vliyaniye gipofiz-adrenalovoy sistemy na immunogenez u belykh myshey (The influence of the hypophyseal-adrenal system on immunogenesis in white mice). In *Sovremennyye problemy immunologii i immunopatologii* (Current problems of immunology and immunopathology), 59–75. Leningrad.

Korneva, E. A. 1961. O roli simpato-adrenalovoy sistemy v regulyatsii protsessa immunogeneza (On the role of the sympathoadrenal system in the regulation of the process of immunogenesis). *Fiziol. Zhurn. SSSR* 49(1):1298–1305.

_____. 1964. O podkorkovoy regulyatsii immunologicheskikh protsessov (On the subcortical regulation of immune processes). In *Ocherki evolyutsii nervnoy deyatel'nosti* (Outlines of the evolution of nervous activity), 102–13. Leningrad.

_____. 1966. K voprosu funktsional'noy organizatsii zon gipotalamusa, preimushchestvenno svyazannykh s regulyatsiyey immunologicheskikh reaktsiy (On the problem of the functional organization of areas of the hypothalamus, primarily involved in the regulation of immune reactions). In *Tez. dokladov II Vsesoyuznoy konferentsii po voprosam fizio-*

logii vegetativnoy nervnoy sistemy (Proceedings of the second all-Union conference on problems of the physiology of the vegetative nervous system), 94–95. Yerevan.

———. 1969. K voprosu o funktsional'noy organizatsii zon mozga, svyazannykh s regulyatsiyey produktsii antitel (On the problem of the functional organization of brain areas involved in the regulation of antibody production). In *Tsentral'nyye mekhanizmy vegetativnoy nervnoy sistemy* (Central mechanisms of the vegetative nervous system), 241–49. Yerevan.

———. 1982. Urovni regulyatsii immunnogo gomeostaza (Levels of regulation of immune homeostasis). In *Materialy dokladov III Vesesoyuznogo simpoziuma "Regulyatsiya immunnogo gomeostaza"* (Proceedings of the third all-Union symposium "The regulation of immune homeostasis"), 19–21. Leningrad.

Korneva, E. A., and Khay, L. M. 1961a. O roli simpato-adrenalovoy sistemy v regulyatsii protsessa immunogeneza (On the role of the sympathoadrenal system in the regulation of the process of immunogenesis). *Fiziol. Zhurn. SSSR* 47(10):1298–1305.

———. 1961b. Ob uchastii simpato-adrenalovoy sistemy i nekotorykh otdelov gipotalamusa v regulyatsii protsessa immunogeneza (On the participation of the sympathoadrenal system and some sections of the hypothalamus in the regulation of the process of immunogenesis). In *Tez. i ref. dokladov 1-go Vsesoyuzno soveshch. po vopr. fiziologii vegetativnoy nervnoy sistemy i mozzhechka* (Proceedings of the first all-Union conference on problems of the physiology of the vegetative nervous system and the cerebellum), 107–8. Yerevan.

———. 1963. Vliyaniye razrusheniya uchastkov gipotalamicheskoy oblasti na protsess immunogeneza (The effect of destruction of segments of the hypothalamic region on the process of immunogenesis). *Fiziol. Zh. SSSR* 49(1):42–48.

———. 1964. O roli simpato-adrenalovoy sistemy i nekotorykh otdelov gipotalamusa v regulyatsii protsessa immunogeneza (On the role of the sympathoadrenal system and some parts of the hypothalamus in the regulation of the process of immunogenesis). In *Voprosy fiziologii vegetativnoy nervnoy sistemy i mozzhechka* (Problems of the physiology of the vegetative nervous system and the cerebellum), 352–56. Yerevan.

———. 1966. O vliyanii razlichnykh struktur mezhutochnogo mozga na protsess obrazovaniya antitel (On the influence of various structures of the diencephalon on the process of antibody formation). In *Tez. dokladov IX Mezhdunar. kongr. po mikrobiologii* (Proceedings of the ninth international congress on microbiology), 612–13. Moscow.

———. 1967. O vliyanii razdrazheniya razlichnykh struktur mezhutochnogo mozga na protekaniye immunologicheskikh reaktsiy (On the influ-

ence of stimulation of various structures of the diencephalon on the course of immune reactions). *Fiziol. Zhurn. SSSR* 53(1):42–47.

Korneva, E. A., and Potin, V. V. 1970. Vliyaniye povrezhdeniya yader zadnego gipotalamusa na tireoidnuyu i ekzoftal'micheskuyu aktivnost' gipofiza krolikov (The influence of damage to the nuclei of the posterior hypothalamus on the thyroid and exophthalmic activity of the hypophysis of rabbits). *Fiziol. Zhurn. SSSR* 56(2):159–64.

Korneva, E. A., and Shekoyan, V. A. 1982. *Regulyatsiya zashchitnykh funktsiy organizma* (The regulation of the defense functions of the organism). Leningrad-Nauka.

Korneva, E. A.; Ogurtsov, R. P.; Zubzhitskiy, Yu. N.; and Klimenko, V. M. 1969. Vliyaniye povrezhdeniya gipotalamusa na immunologicheskiye pokazateli pri "indutsirovannom" ottorzhenii autotransplanta (The influence of damage to the hypothalamus on the immunologic indexes in "induced" rejection of an autotransplant). In *DAN SSSR* (Proceedings of the Academy of Sciences of the USSR), 186(1):215–18.

Korneva, E. A.; Klimenko, V. M.; and Tsvetkova, I. P. 1971. K morfofunktsional'noy kharakteristike struktur zadnego gipotalamusa (On the morphological characteristics of the structures of the posterior hypothalamus). In *Tez. dokladov III Vsesoyuznoy konferentsii po fiziologii vegetativnoy nervnoy sistemy* (Proceedings of the third all-Union conference on the physiology of the vegetative nervous system), 112–13. Yerevan.

Kostinskiy, D. D. 1975. Immunodepressivnoye deystviye muzhskogo polovogo gormona u krys v neonatal'nom periode (The immunodepressive effect of the male sex hormone in rats in the neonatal period). In *Neyrogumoral'naya i farmakologicheskaya korrektsiya immunologicheskikh reaktsiy v eksperimente i klinike. Tez. dokladov* (Neurohumoral and pharmacologic correction of immune reactions under experimental and clinical conditions. Proceedings), 37–38. Leningrad.

Kostyuk, P. G. 1960. *Mikroelektrodnaya tekhnika* (Microelectrode technique). Kiev.

Kozlov, V. A. 1980. Gumoral'no-kletochnyye urovni regulyatsii osnovnykh etapov antitelogeneza (Humoral cellular levels of regulation of the main stages of antibody formation. Dissertation). Moscow.

Kozlov, V. K. 1968. Rol' vegetativnoy nervnoy sistemy v mekhanizmakh anafilakticheskikh reaktsiy (The role of the vegetative nervous system in mechanisms of anaphylactic reactions. Dissertation). Moscow.

———. 1973. *Anafilaksiya i vegetativnaya nervnaya sistema* (Anaphylaxis and the vegetative nervous system). Moscow.

Kozlov, V. K., and Tsyrlova, I. G. 1975. Vliyaniye gidrokortizona na vzaimodeystviye kletok timusa i kostnogo mozga myshey roditel'skogo geno-

tipa v organizme F₁-gibridnogo retsipiyenta (The influence of hydrocortisone on the interaction of cells of the thymus and bone marrow in the organism of a F_1-hybrid recipient). In *Neyrogumoral'naya i farmakologicheskaya korrektsiya immunologicheskikh reaktsiy v eksperimente i klinike. Tez.* dokladov (Neurohumoral and pharmacologic correction of immune reactions under experimental and clinical conditions. Proceedings), 32–33. Leningrad.

Kozlov, V. K.; Kolesnikova, S. M.; and Trufakin, V. A. 1974. Vliyaniye kletok timusa, rezistentnykh k deystviyu gidrokortizona, na proliferatsiyu stvolovykh krovetvornykh kletok (The influence of thymus cells, resistant to the effect of hydrocortisone, on the proliferation of truncal hemopoietic cells). In *DAN SSSR* (Proceedings of the Academy of Sciences of the USSR), 216(2):438–40.

Kraskina, N. A., and Gutorova, N. M. 1962. Metodika vyyavleniya Vi-antitel v syvorotkakh s pomoshch'yu reaktsii passivnoy gemagglyutinatsii (The method of detection of Vi-antibodies in serums with the aid of the reaction of passive hemagglutination). In *Immunopatologiya i profilaktika immunnykh kishechnykh infektsiy* (Immunopathology and prophylaxis of immune intestinal infections), 180–86. Moscow.

Krulich, L.; Hejco, E.; Illner, P.; and Read, C. B. 1974. The effects of acute stress on the secretion of LH, FSH, prolactin and GH in the normal male rat, with comments on their statistical evaluation. *Neuroendocrinology* 16:293–311.

Kulikov, M. A. 1968. Kompleks programm analiza impul'snoy bioelektricheskoy aktivnosti na EVM "Minsk-22" (A complex of programs of analysis of pulsed bioelectrical activity on the "Minsk-22" computer). In *Tez. dokladov II soveshch. po probl. avtomaticheskogo analiza biologicheskikh mikrostruktur i protsessov* (Proceedings of the second conference on problems of automatic analysis of biological microstructures and processes), 90–92. Pushchino.

Kurashvili, V. Ye. 1953. O nekotorykh mekhanizmakh protivogrippoznogo immuniteta (On some mechanisms of anti-influenza immunity). *Medical News* 38:33–35.

———. 1955. Techeniye eksperimental'noy grippoznoy infektsii u belykh myshey pri vyklyuchenii nervnykh retseptorov slizistoy obolochki dykhatel'nykh putey i legkikh (The course of experimental influenza infection in white mice upon elimination of nervous receptors of the mucous membrane of the respiratory tracts and lungs). In *Voprosy patogeneza i immunologii virusnykh infektsiy* (Problems of the pathogenesis and immunology of viral infections), 43–52. Leningrad.

Laborit, H. 1975. The purpose of physiopathology. In *Second international congress on pathological physiology*, 221. Praha.

Ladosz, J. 1969. The influence of the autonomic nervous system on phago-cytosis. 8. Changes caused by chronic administration of carbaminocho-line. *Arch. Immunol. Ther. Exp.* 17:466–75.

Laguchev, S. S. 1975. *Gormony i mitoticheskiy tsikl kletki* (Hormones and the mitotic cycle of the cell). Moscow.

Lance, E. M., and Cooper, S. 1970. Effects of cortisol and antilymphocyte serum on lymphoid populations. In *Hormones and immune response*, 73–75, London.

Larson, D., and Tomlinson, L. 1951. Quantitative antibody studies in man. 1. The effect of adrenal insufficiency and cortisone on the level of circula-tion antibodies. *J. Clin. Investig.* 30:1451–55.

Lawley, D. N., and Maxwell, A. E. 1967. *Faktornyy analiz kak statistiches-kiy metod* (Factor analysis as a statistical method). Moscow.

Lebedev, A. N., and Lutskiy, V. A. 1968. Periodichnost' neyronnoy deya-tel'nosti i nekotoryye predpolozheniya o yeye funksional'nom znachenii (The periodicity of neuronal activity and some assumptions concerning its functional significance). In *Statisticheskaya elektrofiziologiya*. Mater-ialy simpoziuma (Statistical electrophysiology. Proceedings of sympo-sium), 2:325–39. Vilnius.

Lee, K.; Laugman, R. E.; Paetkau, V. H.; and Diener, E. 1975. The cellu-lar basis of cortisone-induced immunosuppression of the antibody re-sponse studied by its reversal *in vitro. Cell. Immunol.* 17:405–17.

Leonavichene, L. K. 1981. Elektricheskaya aktivnost' golovnogo mozga i immunologicheskiye reaktsii pri revmaticheskikh protsessakh (The elec-trical activity of the brain and immune responses during rheumatic pro-cesses. Dissertation). Leningrad.

Leonavichene, L. K., and Astrauskas, V. I. 1975. Vzaimosvyaz' mezhdu elektricheskoy aktivnost'yu obrazovaniy golovnogo mozga i immunnymi reaktsiyami pri modelirovanii revmatoidnogo artrita u krolikov s raz-drazhennymi i koagulirovannymi zadnegipotalamicheskimi yadrami (The interrrelation between the electrical activity of brain structures and immune reactions in modeling rheumatoid arthritis in rabbits with stimu-lated and coagulated posterior hypothalamic nuclei. In *Neyrogumoral-'naya i farmakologicheskaya korrektsiya immunologicheskikh reaktsiy v eksperimente i klinike*. Tez. dokladov (Neurohumoral and pharmacolo-gic correction of immune reactions under experimental and clinical con-ditions. Proceedings), 40–41. Leningrad.

Lesniak, M.; Poth, J.; Goreen, P.; and Gavin, J. 1973. Human growth hor-mone radioreceptor assay using cultured human lymphocytes. *Nature* 241:20–22.

Levick, W. R., and Williams, W. C. 1964. Maintained activity of lateral geniculate neurons in darkness. *J. Physiol.* 170:582–97.

Levine, M. A., and Claman, H. N. 1970. Bone marrow and spleen: Dissociation of immunologic properties by cortisone. *Science* 167:1515–17.

Leytes, S. M. 1964. Permisivnaya rol' glyukokortikoidov v protsessakh obmena veshchestv (The permissive role of glucocorticoids in metabolic
processes). In *Gipofiz–kora nadpochechnikov* (Hypophysis–adrenal cortex), 63–71. Kiev.

Lissák, K., and Endröczi, E. 1967. *Neyroendokrinnaya regulyatsiya adap-
tatsionnoy deyatel'nosti* (Neuroendocrine regulation of adaptive activity). Budapest.

Litvak, R. V. 1956. Kompleks fiziologicheskikh reaktsiy organizma na vve-
deniye mikrobov (The complex of physiological reactions of the organism
to the administration of microbes). In *Osnovy immuniteta* (Principles of
immunity), 37–53. Moscow.

Livanov, M. N. 1965. Neyrokibernetika (Neurocybernetics). In *Problemy
sovremennoy neyrofiziologii* (Problems of modern neurophysiology), 37.
Moscow-Leningrad.

————. 1972. *Prostranstvennaya organizatsiya protsessov golovnogo
mozga* (The spatial organization of cerebral processes). Moscow.

London, Ye. S. 1899. O vliyanii udaleniya razlichnykh chastey golovnogo
mozga na immunitet golubey v otnoshenii sibirskoy yazvy (On the influence of the removal of various parts of the brain on the immunity of pigeons with respect to anthrax). *Arkh. Biol. Nauk* 7:177–87.

Lowry, O. H.; Rosebrough, N. J.; Farr, A. L.; and Randal, R. J. 1951.
Protein measurement with the folinphenol reagent. *J. Biol. Chem.*
193:265–75.

Luk'yanenko, V. I.; Flerov, B. A.; and Kuznetsov, S. M. 1962. Rol' vysshikh otdelov tsNS v tormozhenii mestnoy allergicheskoy reaktsii—fenomena Artyusa-Sakharova (The role of the higher parts of the CNS in the
inhibition of a local allergic reaction—the Arthus-Sakharov phenomenon). *Vestn. Moskovsk. Un-ta* 2:24–29.

Lundin, P. M. 1958. Anterior pituitary gland and lymphoid tissue growth.
Acta Endocrinol. 28:5–81.

————. 1960. Effect of hypophysectomy on antibody formation in the rat.
Acta Path. Microbiol. Scand. 48:351–57.

Luparello, T. J.; Stein, M.; and Park, C. D. 1964. Effect of hypothalamic
lesions on rat anaphylaxis. *Amer. J. Physiol.* 207:911–14.

Luria, M. V.; Zappazodi, P.; Dannenberg, A.; and Swartz, I. 1951. Consti-
tutional factors in resistance to infection: The effect of cortisone on the
pathogenesis of tuberculosis. *Science* 113:234.

McIntyre, H. B., and Odell, W. D. 1974. Physiological control of growth
hormone in the rabbit. *Neuroendocrinology* 16:8–21.

MacManus, J. P.; Whitfield, J. F.; and Yondale, T. 1971. Stimulation by epinephrine of adenyl cyclase activity, cyclic AMP formation, DNA synthesis and cell proliferation in populations of rat thymic lymphocytes. *J. Cell. Physiol.* 77:103–16.

Maestroni, G. J. M.; Pierpaoli, W.; and Zinkernagel, R. M. 1982. Immunoreactivity of long lived H-2 incompatible irradiation chimeras ($H-2^d \rightarrow H-2^b$). *Immunology* 46:253–60.

Magayeva, S. V. 1979. Immunodefitsitnoye sostoyaniye pri eksperimental'-noy patologii gippokampa (The immunodeficient state in experimental hippocampal pathology. Dissertation). Moscow.

Magayeva, S. V.; Borisova, Ye. S.; and Strukova, L. G. 1968. Analiz roli nekotorykh struktur zadnego gipotalamusa v regulyatsii nakopleniya protivomikrobnykh antitel v krovi (Analysis of the role of some structures of the posterior hypothalamus in the regulation of the accumulation of antimicrobic antibodies in the blood). In *Tr. In-ta Norm. i Patol. Fiziol. AMN SSSR* (Proceedings of the Institute of Normal and Pathological Physiology of the Academy of Medical Sciences of the USSR), 11:53–55.

Makara, G. B.; Stark, E.; Palkovits, M.; Révész, T.; and Mihály, K. 1969. Afferent pathways of stressful stimuli: Corticotrophin release after partial deafferentation of the medial basal hypothalamus. *J. Endocrinol.* 44:187–93.

Makarenko, Yu. A., and Frolov, Ye. P. 1972. Oblegchayushchiye i tormozyashchiye effekty emotsional'nykh tsentrov mozga na razvitiye immuniteta i allergii (Facilitating and inhibitory effects of the emotional centers of the brain on the development of immunity and allergy). In *Tez. dokladov 23-go soveshch. po probl. vysshey nervnoy deyatel'nosti* (Proceedings of the twenty-third conference on problems of higher nervous activity), 73–74. Gor'kiy.

Maor, D.; Eylan, E.; and Alexander, P. 1974. Hormones as modulators of ribonuclease activity in lymphoid organs of immunized rats. *Biomed. Express* 21:107–9.

Marakusha, I. G.; Korneva, Ye. A.; and Marat, B. A. 1976. Techeniye vospalitel'nykh protsessov v usloviyakh povrezhdeniya gipotalamicheskikh struktur (The course of inflammatory processes under conditions of damage to the hypothalamic structures). In *Ranniye proyavleniya tkanevoy nesovmestimosti. Tez. dokladov* (Early manifestations of tissue incompatibility. Proceedings), 62. Moscow.

Marat, B. A. 1971. Reaktivnost' leykotsitov perifericheskoy krovi u krolikov s elektricheskim povrezhdeniyem gipotalamusa i izmeneniyem protsessa produktsii antitel (The reactivity of leukocytes of the peripheral

blood in rabbits with electrical injury of the hypothalamus and change in the process of antibody production). In *Infektsionnaya i neinfektsionnaya immunologiya*. Tez. dokladov konferentsii molodykh uchenykh (Infectious and noninfectious immunology. Proceedings of the conference of young scientists), 88–90. Moscow.

————. 1973. Vliyaniye tsentral'nykh kholinolitikov na pervichnyy immunnyy otvet u krolikov (The effect of central cholinolytics on the primary immune response in rabbits). *Byull. Eksperim. Biol. I Med.* 76(8):97–99.

————. 1975. K analizu vliyaniya nekotorykh neyrotropnykh farmakologicheskikh soyedineniy na techeniye pervichnogo immunnogo otveta (On the analysis of the effect of some neurotropic pharmacologic compounds on the course of the primary immune response). In *Neyrogumoral'naya i farmakologicheskaya korrektsiya immunologicheskikh reaktsiy v eksperimente i klinike*. Tez. dokladov (Neurohumoral and pharmacologic correction of immune reactions under experimental and clinical conditions. Proceedings), 46. Leningrad.

March, J. T.; Lavender, J. F.; Chang, S.; and Rasmussen, A. F. 1963. Poliomyelitis in monkeys: Decreased susceptibility after avoidance stress. *Science* 140:1414–15.

Marchuk, P. D. 1956. O vliyanii tsentral'noy nervnoy sistemy na zashchitnyye reaktsii organizma (On the influence of the central nervous system on the protective reactions of the organism). In *Osnovy immuniteta* (Principles of immunity), 3:69–77. Moscow.

Markov, Kh. M. 1966. Izmeneniya EEG pri sensibilizatsii i anafilakticheskom shoke (Changes in the electroencephalogram in sensitization and anaphylactic shock). In *Reaktivnost'*. Materialy konferentsii (Reactivity. Proceedings of conference), 50–51. Moscow.

Maros, T.; Kovács, A.; Mody, E.; and Lázár, L. 1960. Izmeneniya belkovykh fraktsiy krovi posle chastichnoy dekortikatsii i povrezhdeniya nervnykh obrazovaniy mozgovogo stvola (gipotalamus, setchatoye obrazovaniye) (Changes in the protein fractions of the blood after partial decortication and damage to the neural structures of the brain stem—the hypothalamus, the reticular formation). In *Tezisy dokladov konferentsii rumynskikh fiziologov* (Proceedings of the conference of Romanian physiologists), 93–94. Bucharest.

Mashkovskiy, M. D. 1956. Farmakologicheskiye svoystva aminazina i drugikh preparatov fenotiazinovogo ryada (Pharmacologic properties of chlorpromazine and other drugs of the phenothiazine series). *Zhurn. Nevropatol. I Psikhiat.* 56(2):81–94.

Mats-Rossinskaya, V. S. 1957. O roli tsentral'noy nervnoy sistemy v mekhanizme anafilaksii (On the role of the central nervous system in the mechanism of anaphylaxis. Dissertation). Khar'kov.

Mednieks, M. I., and Danute, J. S. 1975. *In vitro* regulation of the immune response by cyclic AMP and a thymic extract. *Immunol. Commun.* 4:99–110.

Medvedev, V. M. 1957. O mekhanizme deystviya virusa grippa na verkhniy sheynyy simpaticheskiy uzel (On the mechanism of action of the influenza virus on the superior cervical sympathetic ganglion). In *O mekhanizmakh deystviya mikrobov na nervnuyu sistemu* (Mechanisms of the action of microbes on the nervous system), 62–67. Moscow.

Meites, J.; Mueller, G. P.; Chen, H. J.; Chen, H. T.; and Dibbot, J. A. 1974. Hypothalamic control of release of TSH, GH and prolactin in the rat. In *Twenty-sixth international congress of physiological science*, 1:93–94. New Delhi.

Melikhova, M. A., and Shul'gina, G. I. 1966. Issledovaniye "spontannoy" impul'snoy aktivnosti neyronov kory bol'shogo mozga krolika (Investigation of the "spontaneous" impulse activity of neurons of the cerebral cortex of rabbits). *Zh. Vyssh. Nervn. Deyat. Im. I. P. Pavlova* 16(2):328–35.

Mel'nikov, V. N. 1954. Vliyaniye medikamentoznogo vozbuzhdeniya TsNS na techeniye bryushnotifoznoy toksikoinfektsii u belykh myshey i nakopleniye agglyutininov pri revaktsinatsii u krolikov (The influence of medicinal stimulation of the CNS on the course of typhoidal toxic infection in white mice and the accumulation of agglutinins upon revaccination in rabbits). *Zhurn. Mikrobiol, Epidemiol., Immunobiol.* 25(7):33–38.

Menitskiy, D. N. 1964. Veroyatnostnyy i ekologicheskiy podkhody v izuchenii deyatel'nosti nervnoy sistemy (The probability and ecological approaches in the study of the activity of the nervous system). In *Ocherki evolyutsii nervnoy deyatel'nosti* (Outline of the evolution of nervous activity), 145–54. Leningrad.

Meshalova, A. N. 1958. Vliyaniye kortizona na protsessy immunogeneza. Soobshch. I. Vliyaniye kortizona na obrazovaniye antitel i fagotsitoz (The influence of cortisone on processes of immunogenesis. First communication. The influence of cortisone on the formation of antibodies and on phagocytosis). *Zhurn. Mikrobiol., Epidemiol., Immunobiol.* 29(10):57–62.

——. 1959. Vliyaniye kortizona na protsessy immunogeneza. Soobshch. II. Immunologicheskiye sdvigi pod vliyaniyem kortizona u immunizirovannykh krolikov (The influence of cortisone on processes of immuno-

genesis. Rept. 2. Immunologic shifts under the influence of cortisone in immunized rabbits). *Zhurn. Mikrobiol., Epidemiol., Immunobiol.* 30(1):11–13.

———. 1961. Vliyaniye kortizona na protsessy immunogeneza. Soobshch. V. Zavisimost' immunologicheskikh reaktsiy organizma ot dozy i vremeni vvedeniya steriodnykh gormonov (The influence of cortisone on processes of immunogenesis. Rept. 5. The dependence of immune reactions of the organism on the dosage and time of injection of steroid hormones). *Zhurn. Mikrobiol., Epidemiol., Immunol.* 32(7):92–97.

Meshalova, A. N., and Fryazinova, I. B. 1960. Vliyaniye kortizona na protsessy immunogeneza. Soobshch. IV. Sravnitel'noye izucheniye reaktivnosti organizma pod vliyaniyem razlichnykh steroidnykh gormonov (The influence of cortisone on processes of immunogenesis. Rept. 4. Comparative study of the reactivity of the organism under the influence of various steroid hormones). *Zhurn. Mikrobiol., Epidemiol., Immunobiol.* 31(6):23–29.

Metcalf, D. 1969. Cortisone action on serum colony-stimulating factor and bone marrow *in vitro* colony-forming cells. In *Proc. Soc. Exp. Biol. Med.*, 391.

Mikaelyan, M. G.; Arutyunyan, V. M.; and Stepanyan, M. S. 1972a. Antiteloobrazovatel'naya funktsiya u krolikov v zavisimosti ot funktsional'-nogo sostoyaniya shchitovidnoy zhelezy (The antibody formation function in rabbits depending on the functional state of the thyroid gland). *Uch. Zap. Yerevanskogo Un-ta Yestestv. Nauk* 2(120):101–5.

Mikaelyan, M. G.; Sakanyan, S. Sh.; Tevosyan, E. Ye.; and Shakhbazyan, P. T. 1972b. Ob uchastii shchitovidnoy zhelezy v formirovanii immunologicheskoy radiorezistentnosti (The participation of the thyroid gland in the formation of immune radiation resistance). In *Trudy nauch. obshchestva endokrinologov Armenii*, 1:68–72. Yerevan.

Mikhaylov, V. V., and Shakharova, G. G. 1969. K mekhanizmu uchastiya timusa v protsessakh prizhivleniya svezhikh gomotransplantatov kozhi u krysyat rannego postnatal'nogo vozrasta i ottorzheniye ikh v boleye pozdnem periode (The mechanism of participation of the thymus in processes of acceptance of fresh homotransplants of skin in rats of early postnatal age and their rejection at a later period). In *Patofiziologiya infektsionnogo protsessa i allergii* (Pathophysiology of infectious processes and allergy), 163–74. Saratov.

Mikhaylov, V. V.; Astaf'yeva, N. T.; and Solov'yeva, V. Ya. 1970. Ob uchastii zadnikh yader gipotalamusa v mekhanizme razvitiya eksperimental'nogo allergicheskogo entsefalita i postdifteriynogo polinevrita (The participation of the posterior hypothalamic nuclei in the mechanism

of the development of experimental allergic encephalitis and postdiphtherial polyneuritis). *Byull. Eksper. Biol. I Med.* 35(2):32–35.

Mikhaylova, A. A. 1981. Gumoral'nyye faktory kostnogo mozga, reguliruyushchiye antitelogenez (Humoral factors of the bone marrow, which regulate antibody formation). In *Itogi nauki i tekhniki. Immunologiya. Mediatory immunnoy sistemy* (Advances in science and technology. Immunology. Mediators of the immune system), 9:110–43.

Mikhaylova, N. V. 1953. Issledovaniye biologicheskoy aktivnosti adrenokortikotropnogo gormona peredney doli gipofiza (Investigation of the biological activity of the adrenocorticotrophic hormone of the anterior lobe of the hypophysis. In *DAN SSSR* (Proceedings of the Academy of Sciences of the USSR), 88(3):579–82.

Miller, J. F. 1975. Induction of the immune (allergic) response. In *Clinical aspects of immunology*, 447–69. Oxford.

Miller, J. F.; and Cole, L. L. 1967. Resistance of long lived lymphocytes and plasma cells in rat lymph nodes to treatment with prednisone. *J. Exp. Med.* 126:109–25.

Mills, J. H.; Schedl, H. P.; Chen, P. S.; and Bartter, F. P. 1960. The effect of estrogen administration on the metabolism and protein binding of hydrocortisone. *J. Clin. Endocrinol.* 20:515–28.

Mirick, G. S. 1951. The effects of ACTH and cortisone on antibodies on human beings. *Bull. Johns Hopkins Hosp.* 88:332–51.

Moeschlin, S.; Baguena, R.; and Baguena, J. 1952. Cited in Fagraens (1952).

Molomut, N. 1939. The effect of hypophysectomy on immunity and hypersensitivity in rats with a brief description of the operative technique. *J. Immunol.* 37:113–31.

Monayenkov, A. M. 1956. Vliyaniye funktsional'nykh izmeneniy v deyatel'nosti kory bol'shikh polushariy golovnogo mozga na immunologicheskuyu reaktivnost' (The influence of functional changes in the activity of the cerebral cortex on immune reactivity). *Zhurn. Mikrobiol., Epidemiol., Immunobiol.* 27(12):88–91.

———. 1970. Nervnaya trofika i autoimmunologicheskiye protsessy (Neural trophism and autoimmune processes). In *Nervnaya trofika v fiziologii i patologii* (Neural trophism in physiology and pathology), 220–30. Moscow.

Monogenova, L. S., and Solov'yeva, V. Ya. 1969. O vliyanii elektricheskogo razrusheniya zadnikh yader gipotalamusa na kharakter morfologicheskikh izmeneniy v kozhnykh gomotransplantatakh (The effect of electrical destruction of the posterior nuclei of the hypothalamus on the nature of morphological changes in skin homotransplants). In *Physiology of the infectious process and allergy*, 174–77. Saratov.

Moor, P. de. 1965. The binding of radiocortisone on transcortin as measured by gel filtration. *Pflug. Arch.* 285:349–59.

Moor, P. de; Deckx, R.; Raus, J.; and Denef, C. 1963. About the possible influence of transcortin on the catabolism of cortisol in the liver. In *Metabolism*, 12:592–97.

Moore, G. P.; Perkel, D. H.; and Segundo, J. P. 1966. Statistical analysis and functional interpretation of neuronal spike data. *Ann. Rev. Physiol.* 28:493–522.

Morenkov, E. S. 1959. Nervnaya regulyatsiya immuniteta (Neural regulation of immunity). In *Materialy nauchn. studench. konf. Rostovskogo Gos. Un-ta, posvyashch. 40-letiyu VLKSM* (Proceedings of the scientific student conference of Rostov State University in honor of the fortieth anniversary of the Young Communist League), 64–72. Rostov-on-Don.

Morgunov, I. N. 1954. K voprosu o regulyatsii nervnoy sistemoy obrazovaniya antitel (On the regulation of antibody formation by the nervous system). *Med. Zhurn.* 24(1):16–23.

Mountcastle, V. B., and Powell, T. P. 1959a. Central nervous mechanisms subserving position sense and kinesthesis. *Bull. Johns Hopkins Hosp.* 105a:173–200.

————. 1959b. Neural mechanisms subserving cutaneous sensibility with special reference to the role of afferent inhibition in sensory perception and discrimination. *Bull. Johns Hopkins Hosp.* 105:201–32.

Murphy, J. T., and Renaud, L. P. 1968. Inhibitory interneurons in the ventromedial nucleus of the hypothalamus. *Brain Res.* 9:385–89.

Mustárdy, L.; Kiss, L.; and Karády, S. 1954. Die Rolle der höheren Nervenfunktion im Mechanismus der Antikörperproduktion. *Acta Physiol. Acad. Sci. Hung.* 6:3–43.

Nagareda, C. S. 1954. Antibody formation and the effect of X-radiation on circulating antibody levels in the hyophysectomized rat. *J. Immunol.* 73(2):88–94.

Nakayama, H.; Nishioka, S.; Otsuka, T.; and Aikawa, S. 1966. Statistical dependency between interspike intervals of spontaneous activity in thalamic lemniscal neurons. *J. Neurophysiol.* 29:921–34.

Nakayama, T.; Eisenman, J. S.; and Hardy, J. D. 1961. Single unit activity of the anterior hypothalamus during local heating. *Science* 134:560–61.

Narushevichus, E. V., and Maginskis, V. A. 1966. Fluktuatsii mezhspaykovykh intervalov u avtoneyronov (The fluctuation of interspike intervals in autoneurons). In *Dinamika neyronnykh setey* (The dynamics of neuronal nets), 67–71. Vilnius.

Nasonov, D. N. 1959. Mestnaya reaktsiya protoplazmy i rasprostranyayushcheyesya vozbuzhdeniye (Local reaction of protoplasm and spreading excitation). Moscow-Leningrad.

Nauta, J. H. 1963. Central nervous organization and endocrine motor system. In *Advances in neuroendocrinology*, 5–21. Urbana.

Nauta, W. J. 1960. Limbic system and hypothalamus: Anatomic aspects. *Physiol. Rev.* 40:102–4.

Nebylitsyn, V. D. 1960. *Voprosy psikhologii* (Problems of psychology), no. 4. Moscow.

_____. 1963. *Tipologicheskiye osobennosti vysshey nervnoy deyatel'nosti cheloveka* (Typological characteristics of human higher nervous activity), no. 3. Moscow.

Nesterenko, K. A. 1958. K voprosu o vliyanii funktsional'nogo sostoyaniya TsNS na immunologicheskiye reaktsii (The influence of the functional state of the CNS on immune reactions). In *Materialy 2-go plenuma Sibirskogo fil. Vsesoyuznoy Obshch-va Patofiziologov* (Proceedings of the second plenary session of the Siberian branch of the All-Union Society of Pathophysiologists), 29–32. Chita.

Newson, S. E., and Darrach, M. 1954. The effect of cortisone acetate on the production of circulating hemolytic antibodies in the mouse. *Canad. J. Biochem. Physiol.* 32:372–82.

Nicol, T., and Belbey, D. L. J. 1960. The effect of various steroids on the phagocytic activity of the reticuloendothelial system. In *Reticuloendothelial structure and function*, 301–20. New York.

Northe, R. 1971. The action of cortisone acetate on cell-mediated immunity to infection. *J. Exp. Med.* 134:1485–1500.

Ohguri, M. 1935. Effect of excluding splanchnic nerves or suprarenal medulla upon hyperglycemia due to anaphylactic shock in dogs. *Tohuku J. Exp. Med.* 25:445–53.

Orlova, L. N. 1958. Deystviye nespetsificheskikh razdrazhiteley na vyrabotku antitel pri immunizatsii zhivotnykh palochkoy koklyusha (The effect of nonspecific stimuli on the development of antibodies in the immunization of animals with whooping-cough bacillus). In *Sbornik studencheskikh rabot Rostovskogo Meditsinskogo Instituta* (Collection of students' works of Rostov Medical Institute), 1:35–36. Rostov-on-Don.

Overall, J. E., and Williams, C. M. 1961. Models for medical diagnosis. *Behav. Sci.* 6:134–41.

Oyvin, I. A., and Sergeyev, Yu. V. 1956. O reflektornom mekhanizme vyrabotki antitel (The reflex mechanism of antibody development). *Zhurn. Mikrobiol., Epidemiol., Immunobiol.* 27(3):98–102.

Palant, B. L.; Oleynikova, Ye. A.; Fintiktinova, R. P.; and Mitel'man, P. M. 1955. Rol' tormozheniya i vozbuzhdeniya TsNS v razvitii nekotorykh infektsiy i immuniteta (The role of inhibition and excitation of the CNS in the development of some infections and immunity). *Zhurn. Mikrobiol., Epidemiol., Immunobiol.* 26(5):53–56.

Pankov, Yu. A., and Usvatova, I. Ya. 1965. Flyurometricheskiy metod opredeleniya 11-oksikortikosteroidov v plazme pericheskoy krovi (The fluorometric method of determination of 11-oxycorticosteroids in the peripheral blood). In *Metody issledovaniya nekotorykh gormonov i mediatorov. Tr. po novoy apparature i metodikam* (Methods of investigation of some hormones and mediators. Publications on new instrumentation and methods), 3:137–45. Moscow.

Park, B. H.; Beck, N. P.; and Good, R. A. 1974. Changes in the levels of cyclic AMP in human leukocytes during phagocytosis. In *Cyclic AMP, cell growth and immune response,* 284–89. Berlin.

Pastukhov, N. A. 1975. Vliyaniye emotsional'nykh stressorov na funktsiyu shchitovidnoy zhelezy (The influence of emotional stressors on the function of the thyroid gland). *Probl. Endokrinol.* 21(2):15–19.

Pel'ts, D. G. 1955. Rol' kory bol'shikh polushariy mozga v izmenenii fagotsitarnoy aktivnosti leykotsitov krovi zhivotnykh pri nanesenii im elektrokozhnykh razdrazheniy (The role of the cerebral cortex in the change of the phagocytic activity of blood leukocytes of animals upon application of electrocutaneous stimulation). *Byull. Eksper. Biol. I Med.* 40(9):55–58.

Perkel, D. H.; Schulman, J. H.; Bullock, T. H.; Moore, J. P.; and Segundo, J. P. 1964. Pacemaker neurons: Effects of regularly spaced synaptic input. *Science* 145:61–63.

Petrov, R. V. 1976. *Immunologiya i immunogenetika* (Immunology and immunogenetics). Moscow.

Petrov, R. V., and Zaretskaya, Yu. M. 1965. *Transplantatsionnyy immunitet i radiatsionnyye khimery* (Transplantation immunity and radiation chimeras). Moscow.

Petrov, R. V.; Khaitov, R. M.; Bezin, G. I.; and Rachkov, S. M. 1975. Regulyatornoye vliyaniye gipofiz-adrenalovoy sistemy na migratsiyu stvolovykh kletok T- i B- limfotsitov: vozdeystviye adrenalektomii, AKTG i gidrokortizona (The regulatory effect of the hypophyseal-adrenal system on the migration of stem cells of T- and B-lymphocytes: The effect of adrenalectomy, adrenocorticotrophic hormone, and hydrocortisone). In *Neyrogumoral'naya i farmakologicheskaya korrektsiya immunologsicheskikh reaktsiy v eksperimente i klinike. Tez. dokladov* (Neurohumoral and pharmacologic correction of immune reactions under experimental and clinical conditions. Proceedings), 52–53. Leningrad.

Petrov, R. V.; Novikov, V. I.; and Mikhaylova, A. A. 1981. Vklyucheniye sinteza antitel v "molchashchey" populyatsii antiteloprodutsentov pod vliyaniyem kostnomozgovogo mediatora—SAP (The startup of antibody synthesis in a "silent" antibody-producer population under the influence

of the bone-marrow mediator SAP). In *DAN SSSR* (Proceedings of the academy of sciences of the USSR), 258(5):1258–60.

Petrovskiy, I. N. 1961. Voprosy nervnoy regulyatsii reaktsiy immuniteta. Soobshch. I. Vliyaniye razdrazheniya razlichnykh uchastkov golovnogo mozga na titr agglyutininov (Problems of the nervous regulation of reactions of immunity. Rept. 1. The influence of stimulation of various sections of the brain on the titer of agglutinins). *Zhurn. Mikrobiol., Epidemiol., Immunobiol.* 32(7):103–8.

Pierpaoli, W. 1981. Integrated phylogenetic and ontogenetic evolution of neuroendocrine and identity-defense, immune function. In *Psychoneuroimmunology*, ed. R. Ader, 575–606. New York: Academic Press.

Pierpaoli, W., and Sorkin, E. 1967. Relationship between thymus and hypophysis. *Nature* 215:834–37.

———. 1968a. Cited in Pierpaoli et al. (1969).

———. 1968b. Effect of gonadectomy on the peripheral lymphatic tissue of neonatally thymectomized mice. *Brit. J. Exp. Path.* 49:288–93.

———. 1968c. Hormones and immunological capacity. 1. Effect of heterologous anti-growth hormone (ASTH) antiserum on thymus and peripheral lymphatic tissue in mice. Induction of a wasting syndrome. *J. Immunol.* 101:1036–43.

———. 1969a. Effect of growth hormone and antigrowth hormone on the lymphatic tissue and the immune response. *Antibiot. Chemother.* 15:122–34.

———. 1969b. A study on antipituitary serum. *Immunology* 16:311–18.

Pierpaoli, W.; Baroni, E.; Fabris, N.; and Sorkin, E. 1969. Hormones and immunological capacity. 2. Reconstitution of antibody production in hormonally deficient mice by somatotropic hormone, thyrotropic hormone and thyroxine. *Immunology* 16:217–30.

Plescia, O. J.; Yamamoto, I.; and Shimamura, T. 1975. Cyclic AMP and immune responses: Changes in the splenic level of cyclic AMP during the response of mice to antigen. In *Proc. Nat. Acad. Sci. USA*, 72:888–91.

Pletsityy, D. F., and Magayeva, S. V. 1970. O regulyatsii immunogeneza strukturami gippokampa (The regulation of immunogenesis by hippocampal structures). In *DAN SSSR* (Proceedings of the Academy of Sciences of the USSR), 194(1):232–33.

Pletsityy, D. F., and Monayenkov, A. M. 1963. Tip nervnoy sistemy loshadey i effektivnost' ikh giperimmunizatsii (The type of nervous system of horses and the effectiveness of their hyperimmunization). In *Tez. dokladov 19-go soveshch. po probl. vysshey nervnoy deyatel'nosti* (Proceedings of the nineteenth conference on problems of higher nervous activity), 193–94. Moscow-Leningrad.

Plokhinskiy, N. A. 1970. *Biometriya* (Biometry). Moscow.

Podpolzin, A. A. 1963. Deystviye immunykh kompleksov na verkhniy sheynyy simpaticheskiy uzel (The effect of immune complexes on the superior cervical sympathetic ganglion). *Vestn. AMN SSSR* 11:25–28.

Poggio, G. F., and Mountcastle, V. B. 1963. The functional properties of ventrobasal thalamic neurons studied in unanesthetized monkeys. *J. Neurophysiol.* 26:775.

Poggio, G. F., and Viernstein, L. J. 1964. Time series analysis of impulse sequences of thalamic somatic sensory neurones. *J. Neurophysiol.* 27:517–45.

Polenov, A. L. 1971. *Gipotalamicheskaya neyrosekretsiya* (Hypothalamic neurosecretion). Leningrad.

Polishchuk, I. A., and Vashetko, V. A. 1958. Vliyaniye aminazina i serpazila na obmennyye protsessy pri psikhicheskikh zabolevaniyakh (The effect of chlorpromazine and reserpine on metabolic processes in mental disease). *Zhurn. Nevropatol. I Psikhiat.* 58(10):1153–64.

Poltavchenko, G. M. 1982. Uchastiye adrenergicheskikh mekhanizmov v regulyatsii protsessov immunogeneza (The participation of adrenergic mechanisms in the regulation of processes of immunogenesis. Dissertation). Leningrad.

Polushkin, B. V. 1971. Allergoidnyye reaktsii (Allergoid reactions). *Usp. Sovrem. Biol.* 71(2):253–71.

Polyak, A. I. 1968. O vtorichnoy immunologicheskoy reaktsii na fone razrusheniya razlichnykh yader mezhutochnogo mozga (Secondary immune reaction after destruction of various nuclei of the diencephalon). In *Mekhanizmy nekotorykh patologicheskikh protsessov* (Mechanisms of certain pathological processes), 2:429–37. Rostov-on-Don.

———. 1969. Nekotoryye mekhanizmy regulyatsii fenomenov immuniteta (Some mechanisms of the regulation of phenomena of immunity. Dissertation). Perm'.

Polyak, A. I., and Bogdanchikova, V. V. 1967. Model'noye izucheniye tsentral'nykh mekhanizmov antitelogeneza (Model study of the central mechanisms of antibody formation). In *Modelirovaniye, metody izucheniya i eksperimental'naya terapiya patologicheskikh protsessov* (Modeling, methods of study, and experimental therapy of pathological processes), 2:68–72. Moscow.

Polyak, A. I., and Rumbesht, L. M. 1968. Antiteloobrazovaniye pri razlichnykh variantakh immunizatsii na fone vyklyucheniya yader gipotalamusa (Antibody formation with different variants of immunization after elimination of the hypothalamic nuclei). In *Mekhanizmy nekotorykh patologicheskikh protsessov* (Mechanisms of certain pathological processes), 448–57. Rostov-on-Don.

Polyak, A. I., and Zotova, V. V. 1975. K mekhanizmam neyrogumoral'noy regulyatsii autoimmunnogo protsessa v limfoidnoy tkani (Mechanisms of neurohumoral regulation of the autoimmune process in lymphoid tissue). In *Neyrogumoral'naya i farmakologicheskaya korrektsiya immunologicheskikh reaktsiy v eksperimente i klinike*. Tez. dokladov (Neurohumoral and pharmacologic correction of immune reactions under experimental and clinical conditions. Proceedings), 53–54. Leningrad.

Polyak, A. I.; Rumbesht, L. M.; and Sinichkin, A. A. 1969. Sintez antitel na fone elektrokoagulyatsii zadnegipotalamicheskogo yadra gipotalamusa (Synthesis of antibodies after electrocoagulation of the posterior hypothalamic nucleus). *Zhurn. Mikrobiol., Epidemiol., Immunobiol.* 40(3):52–56.

Polyak, A. I.; Zotova, V. V.; Rumbesht, L. M.; Zakharchenko, Ye. P.; Kishkovskaya, O. V.; Mezhova, L. I.; Belovolova, R. A.; and Minakov, V. I. 1970. K patofiziologii regulyatornykh mekhanizmov nekotorykh patologicheskikh reaktsiy (Pathophysiology of regulatory mechanisms of some pathological reactions). In *Materialy V vsesoyuznoy konferentsii patofiziologov* (Proceedings of the fifth all-union conference of pathophysiologists), 630–31. Baku.

Polyak, A. I.; Zotova, V. V.; Rumbesht, L. M.; and Belovolova, R. A. 1974. K uchastiyu vegetativnoy nervnoy sistemy v regulyatsii immunogeneza (The participation of the vegetative nervous system in the regulation of immunogenesis). In *Materialy IV konferentsii patofiziologov Sev. Kavkaza* (Proceedings of the fourth conference of pathophysiologists of the Northern Caucasus), 102–4. Makhachkala.

Polyak, A. I.; Lebedev, K. A.; Ganina, V. Ya.; Chebotareva, G. S.; and Izotova, V. V. 1975. Ob osobennostyakh immunomorfologicheskogo substrata pri vtorichnoy immunizatsii v zavisimosti ot funktsional'nogo sostoyaniya yader gipotalamusa (Characteristics of the immunomorphologic substratum upon secondary immunization in relation to the functional state of the hypothalamic nuclei). *Zhurn. Mikrobiol., Epidemiol., Immunobiol.* 45(10):107–17.

Polyak, A. I.; Rumbesht, L. M.; Druyan, L. E.; and Perelygina, G. M. 1982. O tsentral'nykh mekhanizmakh korrektsii immunologicheskogo otveta, anafilaksii i stolbnyachnoy intoksikatsii (The central mechanisms of correction of the immune response, anaphylaxis, and tetanus intoxication). In *Materialy dokladov III vsesoyuznogo simpoziuma "Regulyatsiya immunnogo gomeostaza"* (Proceedings of the third all-Union symposium "The regulation of immune homeostasis"), 162–64. Leningrad.

Ponomarev, A. V., and Ebert, L. Ya. 1956. Materialy po neyrogumoral'noy regulyatsii immunogeneza (Materials on the neurohumoral regulation of

immunogenesis). In *Osnovy immuniteta* (Principles of immunity), 141–53. Moscow.

Popjak, G. 1940. The pathway of pituitary colloid through the hypothalamus. *J. Pathol. Bacterial.* 51:83–89.

Preobrazhenskiy, N. I., and Yarovitskiy, N. V. 1963. Primeneniye matematicheskikh metodov dlya issledovaniya impul'snoy aktivnosti tsentral'-nykh neyronov mozga (The application of mathematical methods in the investigation of the impulse activity of the central neurons of the brain). *Biofizika* 8:387–93.

Pronin, L. A. 1954. Vliyaniye obrazovaniya oboronitel'nykh uslovnykh refleksov i sryvov VND na sostoyaniye reaktivnosti u krolikov (The influence of the formation of conditioned defense reflexes and of breakdowns of higher nervous activity on the state of reactivity in rabbits). In *Problema reaktivnosti v patologii* (The problem of reactivity in pathology), 217–25. Moscow.

Pytskaya, Ye. G. 1970. Otsenka allergennykh svoystv bakterial'nykh antigenov i proteinov syvorotok po izmeneniyu metabolizma kortizona v pecheni sobak (Evaluation of the allergenic properties of bacterial antigens and serum proteins from the change in cortisone metabolism in the liver of dogs. Dissertation). Moscow.

Pytskiy, V. I. 1954. Cited in Ado (1959).

———. 1969. Nadpochechnikovyye i vnenadpochechnikovyye mekanizmy snabzheniya tkaney kortizonom pri allergii (Adrenal and extra-adrenal mechanisms of supplying the tissues with cortisone during allergy. Dissertation). Moscow.

Pytskiy, V. I.; Orlov, S. M.; Gulyy, Yu. L.; Syusyukin, Yu. P.; Pytskaya, Ye. G.; Donadze, D. S.; Sakandelidze, O. G.; and Tomilets, V. A. 1972. Mekhanizm glyukokortikoidnoy nedostatochnosti pri allergii (The mechanism of glucocorticoid insufficiency during allergy). In *Aktual'-nyye problemy fiziol., biokhim. i patol. endokrinnoy sistemy.* Tez. dokladov (Essential problems of the physiology, biochemistry, and pathology of the endocrine system. Proceedings), 131. Moscow.

Queiroz, J. M.; Oliveira, L. A.; Vasguez, P. L.; and Dias, S. W. 1975. Immunologic phagocytosis by macrophages: Effect of cholinergic drugs and cylic GMP. *Rev. Brasil. Pesguises Med. Biol.* 8:119–23.

Rafika, M. O. 1960. O fiziologicheskom mekhanizme sensibilizatsii (The physiological mechanism of sensitization). In *Tez. dokladov III vsesoyuznoy konferentsii patofiziologov* (Proceedings of the third all-Union conference of pathophysiologists), 138–39. Moscow.

Reilly, R. W.; Thompson, J. S.; Bielski, R. K.; and Severson, C. D. 1967. Estradiol-induced wasting syndrome in neonatal mice. *J. Immunol.* 98:321–30.

Repin, I. S. 1969. Peredniy gipotalamus i regulyatsiya temperatury tela (The anterior hypothalamus and the regulation of body temperature). In *Tsentral'nyye mekhanizmy vegetativnoy nervnoy sistemy* (Central mechanisms of the vegetative nervous system), 320-27. Yerevan.

Roberts, S., and White, A. 1951. The influence of the adrenal cortex on antibody production *in vitro. Endocrinol.* 48:741-43.

Rodieck, R. W.; Kiang, N. Y. S.; and Gerstein, G. L. 1962. Some quantitative methods for the study of spontaneous activity of single neurons. *Biophys. J.* 2:351-68.

Rodshteyn, O. A.; Konovalov, G. V.; Khay, L. M.; Korneva, Ye. A.; and Shkhinek, E. K. 1974. Miyelinotoksicheskiye antitela v syvorotkakh krolikov bol'nykh EAP (Myelotoxic antibodies in serums of rabbits afflicted with EAP). *Vestn. AMN SSSR* 11:46-49.

Rose, B. 1959. Hormones and allergic responses. In *Mechanisms of hypersensitivity.* Henry Ford Hospital international symposium, 599-612. Boston-Toronto-London.

Rozen, V. B. 1973. Nekotoryye aktual'nyye aspekty dinamiki steroidnykh gormonov (Some essential aspects of the dynamics of steroid hormones). In *Fiziologiya cheloveka i zhivotnykh* (Physiology of man and animals), 2:49-107. Moscow.

Rozen, V. B., and Pankova, S. S. 1971. Dal'neysheye izucheniye voprosa o roli gipofiza v regulyatsii svyazyvayushchey sposobnosti transkortina (kortikoidsvyazyvayushchego globulina) u morskoy svinki (Further study of the role of the hypophysis in the regulation of the binding capacity of transcortin [corticoid-binding globulin] in guinea pigs). *Probl. Endokrinol.* 17(1):70-74.

Rozen, V. B.; Volchek, A. G.; Strokova, I. G.; and Belenev, Yu. 1973. O roli gipotalamo-gipfizarnoy sistemy v regulyatsii urovnya transkortina v plazme krys (The role of the hypothalamohypophyseal system in the regulation of the transcortin level in the plasma of rats). *Probl. Endokrinol.* 19(2):58-63.

Ruben, L. N., and Vaughan, M. R. 1974. The effect of hydrocortisone on the sheep red cell response in adult *Xenopus lacvis*, the South African clawed toad. *J. Exp. Zool.* 190:229-35.

Rumbesht, L. M. 1970. Vliyaniye zadnego gipotalamicheskogo yadra na formirovaniye immunologicheskikh reaktsiy (The influence of the posterior hypothalamic nucleus on the development of immune reactions). In *Mekhanizmy nekotorykh patologicheskikh protsessov* (Mechanisms of certain pathological processes), 3:363-76. Rostov-on-Don.

Rumbesht, L. M., and Shtokolova, R. A. 1967. K voprosu o roli zandnegipotalamicheskogo yadra v regulyatsii fagotsitarnoy aktivnosti leykotsitov (The role of the posterior hypothalamic nucleus in the regulation of

the phagocytic activity of leukocytes). In *Mekhanizmy nekotorykh pato-logicheskikh protsessov* (Mechanisms of certain pathological processes), 1:22–29. Rostov-on-Don.

Ryzhenkov, V. Ye. 1968. Deystviye tsentral'nykh neyrotropnykh veshchestv na sistemu gipofiz-kora nadpochechnikov pri razlichnykh yeye sostoyan-iyakh (The effect of central neurotropic substances on the hypophyseal-adrenocortical system in its various states. Dissertation). Leningrad.

Saakov, B. A., and Polyak, A. I. 1967. K voprosu o tsentral'nykh mekhan-izmakh immunogeneza (The problem of the central mechanisms of im-munogenesis). In *Mekhanizmy nekotorykh patologicheskikh protsessov* (Mechanisms of certain pathological processes), 1:5–13. Rostov-on-Don.

————. 1968. K tsentral'noy regulyatsii immunogeneza (On the central reg-ulation of immunogenesis). In *Mekhanizmy nekotorykh patologiches-kikh protsessov* (Mechanisms of certain pathological processes), 419–24. Rostov-on-Don.

Saakov, B. A.; Gul'yants, E. S.; Gavrilova, T. M.; and Bardakhch'yan, E. A. 1969. Vliyaniye geparina na gipotalamicheskuyu neyrosekretsiyu i yego rol' v reaktsii sistemy gipofiz-nadpochechnik pri fenomene Shvarts-mana (The influence of heparin on hypothalamic neurosecretion and its role in the reaction of the hypophyseal-adrenal system in the Shwartzman phenomenon). *Farmakol. I Toksikol.* 32(2):172–74.

Saakov, B. A.; Polyak, A. I.; Zotova, V. V.; Rumbesht, L. M.; Zakhar-chenko, Ye. P.; Kishkovskaya, O. V.; Perelygina, T. M.; and Chebotar-eva, T. S. 1976. Neyrogumoral'nyye mekhanizmy formirovaniya im-munologicheskikh i immunopatologicheskikh reaktsiy (Neurohumoral mechanisms of the formation of immune and immunopathological reac-tions). In *Mekhanizmy povrezhdeniya, rezistentnosti, adaptatsii i kom-pensatsii*. Tez. dokladov (Mechanisms of injury, resistance, adaptation, and compensation. Proceedings), 2:279–80. Tashkent.

Sakanyan, S. Sh.; Mamikonyan, R. S.; and Torosyan, S. Ye. 1972a. O roli shchitovidnoy zhelezy v mekhanizme vliyaniya kory golovnogo mozga na postvaktsinal'nyy immunitet pri brutselleze (The role of the thyroid gland in the mechanism of the influence of the cerebral cortex on postvaccina-tion immunity in brucellosis). In *Trudy Nauchn. Obshch-va Endokrino-logov Armenii* (Proceedings of the Scientific Society of Endocrinologists of Armenia), 61:55–60. Yerevan.

Sakanyan, S. Sh.; Mamikonyan, R. S.; Torosyan, S. Ye.; and Aznauryan, A. V. 1972b. O morfo-funktsional'nykh izmeneniyakh nekotorykh en-dokrinnykh zhelez i ikh korrelyatsii u krolikov, immunizirovannykh shtammom 19 (Morph-functional changes of some endocrine glands and their correlation in rabbits immunized with strain 19). In *Trudy Nauchn.*

Obshch-va Endokrinologov Armenii (Proceedings of the Scientific Society of Endocrinologists of Armenia), 1:277–87. Yerevan.

Sakanyan, S. Sh.; Mikaelyan, M. G.; Tevosyan, E. Ye.; and Shakhbazyan, P. T. 1972c. K voprosu o roli shchitovidnoy zhelezy v immunogeneze protiv ospy krolikov (The role of the thyroid gland in immunogenesis against smallpox of rabbits). In *Trudy Nauch. Obshch-va Endokrinologov Armenii* (Proceedings of the Scientific Society of Endocrinologists of Armenia), 1:73–75. Yerevan.

Savchenko, I. G. 1981. K voprosu o nevospriimchivosti k sibirskoy yazve (On the unsusceptibility to anthrax). *Vrach* 5:132–34.

Savchuk, O. Ye. 1952. K voprosu o vliyanii TsNS na obrazovaniye antitel (The influence of the CNS on antibody formation). *Med. Zhurn.* 22(2):64–66.

———. 1955. Uslovnyye refleksy i obrazovaniye antitel (Conditioned reflexes and antibody formation). In *Tr. Odesskogo Un-ta, seriya biol. nauk* (Proceedings of Odessa University, biological sciences series), 145(7):105–10.

Sawa, M.; Maruyama, N.; Hanai, T.; and Koyi, S. 1959. Regulatory influence of amygdaloid nuclei upon the unitary activity in ventromedial nucleus of hypothalamus. *Folia Psychiat. Neurol. Jap.* 13:235–56.

Sawyer, C. H.; Everett, J. W.; and Green, J. D. 1954. The rabbit diencephalon in stereotaxic coordinates. *J. Comp. Neurol.* 101:801–24.

Schellin, U.; Hessalsjo, R.; Paulsen, F.; and Mallyrek, J. 1954. Plasma cell production by pituitary somatotrophic hormone in the adaptation syndrome. *Acta Path. Microbiol. Scand.* 3:503–11.

Schmutzler, W., and Freundt, G. P. 1975. The effect of glucocorticoids and catecholamines on cyclic AMP and allergic histamine release in guinea pig lung. *Intern. Arch. Allergy Appl. Immunol.* 49:209–12.

Schwell, S., and Long, D. A. 1956. A species difference with regard to the effect of cortisone acetate on body weight, y-globulin and circulating antitoxin levels. *J. Hyg.* 54:452–60.

Seal, U. S., and Doe, R. P. 1962. Corticosteroid-binding globulin. 1. Isolation from plasma of diethylstilbestrol-treated men. *J. Biol. Chem.* 237:3136–40.

Selye, H. 1952. *The story of the adaptation syndrome.* Montreal: Acta Medical Publishers.

———. 1972. *Na urovne tselogo organizma* (At the level of the whole organism). Moscow.

Sergeyev, G. A.; Pavlova, L. P.; and Romanenko, A. R. 1968. *Statisticheskiye metody issledovaniya entsefalogramm cheloveka* (Statistical methods of the investigation of human encephalograms). Leningrad.

Sergeyev, P. V.; Seyfulla, R. D.; and Mayskiy, A. I. 1971. *Molekulyarnyye aspekty deystviya steroidnykh gormonov* (Molecular aspects of the effect of steroid hormone). Moscow.

Serov, V. V.; Rabina, E. V.; Khay, L. M.; and Korneva, Ye. A. 1972. Morfologiya immunogo otveta pri razrushenii dorsal'nogo polya gipotalamusa (Morphology of the immune response upon destruction of the dorsal area of the hypothalamus). In *Morfologicheskiye osnovy klinicheskoy i eksperimental'noy patologii* (Morphological principles of clinical and experimental pathology), 33–39. Moscow.

Shannon, A. D., and Jones, M. A. 1974. Influence of corticotrophic and corticosteroid hormones on the output of cells from the popliteal lymph node of the sheep. *Austral. J. Exp. Biol. Med. Sci.* 52:515–25.

Shapiro, A. I. 1957. *Nespetsificheskiy immunitet i yego znacheniye v psikhiatricheskoy i nevrologicheskoy klinike* (Nonspecific immunity and its significance in psychiatric and neurological clinical practice). Leningrad.

Shapovalov, A. I. 1964. Elektrofiziologicheskiye metody izucheniya simpaticheskogo provedeniya (Electrophysiological methods of the study of sympathetic conduction). In *Sovremennyye problemy elektrofiziologichekikh issledovaniy nervnoy sistemy* (Present-day problems of electrophysiological investigations of the nervous system), 50–75. Moscow.

————. 1966. *Kletochnyye mekhanizmy simpaticheskoy peredachi* (Cellular mechanisms of sympathetic transmission). Moscow.

Shargin, S. M., and Povazhenko, A. A. 1974. Sutochnyye ritmy soderzhaniya T- i B-limfotsitov v perifericheskoy krovi cheloveka (Diurnal rhythms in the content of T- and B-lymphocytes in human peripheral blood). In *Adaptatsiya i problemy obshchey patologii* (Adaptation and problems of general pathology), 3:115–16. Novosibirsk.

Shatilova, N. V.; Undritsov, M. I.; Frolov, Ye. P.; Lukicheva, T. I.; and Vinitskaya, Ye. B. 1970. Izucheniye roli mediatorov v razvitii fenomena allergicheskoy al'teratsii leykotsitov pri streptokokkovoy allergii nemedlennogo tipa (The study of the role of mediators in the development of the phenomenon of allergic alteration of leukocytes in streptococcal allergy of the immediate type). In *Materialy V Vsesoyuznoy konferentsii patofiziologii* (Proceedings of the fifth all-Union conference of pathophysiologists), 60–61. Baku.

Shekoyan, V. A. 1975. Rol' otdel'nykh struktur gipotalamusa v regulyatsii monotsitarnoy fagotsitiruyushchey sistemy (The role of individual structures of the hypothalamus in the regulation of the monocytic phagocytizing system). In *Neyrogumoral'naya i farmakologicheskaya korrektsiya immunologicheskikh reaktsiy v eksperimente i klinike*. Tez. dokladov (Neurohumoral and pharmacologic correction of immune reactions un-

der experimental and clinical conditions. Proceedings), 74–75. Leningrad.

_____. 1976. Immunogennost' antigena, svyazannogo s RNK i lizosomnymi fraktsiyami makrofagov krolikov s koagulirovannym zadnim gipotalamusom (Immunogenesis of the antigen bound with ribonucleic acid and lysosomic fractions of macrophages of rabbits with coagulated posterior hypothalamus). *Zhurn. Eksper. I Klinich. Med.* 16(2):12–16.

_____. 1977. Gipotalamus i mononuklearnaya fagotsitiruyushchaya sistema (The hypothalamus and the monunuclear phagocytic system. Dissertation). Leningrad.

Shekoyan, V. A., and Khasman, E. L. 1973. O roli zadnego gipotalamusa v regulyatsii funktsii makrofagov (The role of the posterior hypothalamus in the regulation of the function of macrophages). *Byull. Eksper. Biol. I Med.* 76(8):93–96.

Shekoyan, V. A.; Khasman, E. L.; and Uchitel', I. Ya. 1975. Vliyaniye struktur perednego i zadnego gipotalamusa na zakhvat i perevarivaniye antigena makrofagami i klirens tushi (The influence of the structures of the anterior and posterior hypothalamus on the capture and digestion of antigen by macrophages and the clearance of the carcass). *Zhurn. Mikrobiol., Epidemiol., Immunobiol.* 45(3):131–35.

Shekoyan, V. A.; Krymskiy, A. D.; and Nestayko, G. V. 1976. Poverkhnostnaya struktura krolich'ikh peritoneal'nykh makrofagov pri povrezhdenii gipotalamicheskikh struktur (The surface structure of peritoneal macrophages of rabbits upon injury of hypothalmic structures). *Arkh. Patol.* 1:67–70.

Shekoyan, V. A.; Gevorkyan, M. I.; and Tovmasyan, V. S. 1982. Rol' okoloshchitovidnykh zhelez v immunologicheskikh protsessakh (The role of the parathyroid glands in immune processes). In *Materialy dokladov III Vsesoyuznogo simpoziuma "Regulyatsiya immunnogo gomeostaza"* (Proceedings of the third all-Union symposium "The regulation of immune homeostasis"), 112–13. Leningrad.

Shemerovskaya, T. G. 1974. Eksperimental'nyye issledovaniya deystviya nekotorykh gormonov na kletochnyy i gumoral'nyy immunitet (Experimental investigations of the effect of some hormones on cellular and humoral immunity. Dissertation). Leningrad.

Shemerovskaya, T. G., and Kovaleva, I. G. 1975. Stimulyatsiya somatotropnym gormonom kletochnogo immuniteta i immunologicheskoy pamyati (Stimulation by the somatotropic hormone of cellular immunity and immunologic memory). *Byull. Eksper. Biol. I Med.* 79(5):78–80.

Shepotinovskiy, V. I. 1966. K voprosu o roli gipotalamusa v realizatsii vozdeystviya geterokrovi na mozgovoye veshchestvo nadpochechnika (On

the role of the hypothalamus in the implementation of the effect of heter-oblood on the adrenal medulla). In *Tez. dokladov III ob"yed. nauchn. konf. Rostovskogo Med. In-ta i Nauchno-issled. In-tov* (Proceedings of the third combined scientific conference of the Rostov Medical Institute and Research Institute), 131–32. Rostov-on-Don.

Sherman, J. D.; Adner, M. M.; and Dameshen, W. 1964. Effect of thymec-tomy on golden hamster. 2. Studies of the immune response in thymecto-mized and splenectomized non-wasted animals. *Blood* 23:375–88.

Shkhinek, E. K. 1975a. O funktsional'noy roli zadnego gipotalamiches-kogo polya v realizatsii reaktsiy gipotalamo-gipofizarno-adrenalovoy sis-temy (The functional role of the posterior hypothalamic area in the im-plementation of reactions of the hypothalamohypophyseal-adrenal system). *Probl. Endokrinol.* 21(6):59–65.

———. 1975b. K voprosu o roli glyukokortikoidnykh gormonov v dina-mike razvitiya immunnogo otveta v tselostnom organizme (On the role of glucocorticoid hormones in the dynamics of development of an im-mune response in the intact organism). In *Neyrogumoral'naya i farmako-logicheskaya korrektsiya immunologicheskikh reatksiy v eksperimente i klinike.* Tez. dokladov (Neurohumoral and pharmacologic correction of immune reactions under experimental and clinical conditions. Proceed-ings), 76. Leningrad.

Shkhinek, E. K.; Patalova, V. N.; and Abdullin, G. Z. 1967. Izmeneniya nervnoy regulyatsii endokrinnykh funktsiy pri deystvii ioniziruyushchey radiatsii na organizm (Changes in the nervous regulation of endocrine functions during the action of ionizing radiation on the organism). In *Podkorkovo-stvolovyye funktsii pri deystvii ioniziruyushchey radiatsii na organizm* (Subcortical and brain-stem functions during the action of ionizing radiation on the organism), 70–88. Leningrad.

Shkhinek, E. K.; Tsvetkova, I. P.; and Marat, B. A. 1973. Analiz neyroen-dokrinnykh vliyaniy zadnego gipotalamusa na dinamiku spetsificheskikh zashchitnykh reaktsiy u krolikov (Analysis of neuroendocrine influences of the posterior hypothalamus on the dynamics of specific protective re-actions in rabbits). *Fiziol. Zh. SSSR* 59(2):228–36.

Shkhinek, E. K.; Marat, B. A.; and Tsvetkova, I. P. 1974. Izmeneniya funk-tsii gipofiz-adrenalovoy sistemy v dinamike razvitiya immunnogo otveta (Changes in the function of the hypophyseal-adrenal system in the dynamics of the development of an immune response). In *Materialy IV konferentsii patofiziologov Sev. Kavkaza* (Proceedings of the fourth conference of pathophysiologists of the Northern Caucasus), 249–50. Makhachkala.

Shkhinek, E. K.; Dostoyevskaya, L. P.; Fomicheva, Ye. Ye.; and Lesni-kova, M. P. 1982a. Glyukokortikoidnyye gormony i spetsificheskiye

zashchitnyye reaktsii v tselostnom organizme (Glucocorticoid hormones and specific defense reactions in the intact organism). In *Tezisy dokladov III Vsesoyuznogo s"yezda patofiziologov "Povrezhdeniye i regulyatornyye protsessy organizma"* (Proceedings of the third all-Union conference of pathophysiologists "Damage and regulatory processes of the organism"), 99. Tbilisi.

Shkhinek, E. K.; Korneva, Ye. A.; Stark, E.; Ach, Zs.; Abavari, K.; Szalai, K.; and Fiok, J. 1982b. Glyukokortikoidnyye gormony i immunnyy otvet (The glucocorticoid hormones and the immune response). In *Materialy dokladov III Vsesoyuznogo simpoziuma "Regulyatsiya immunnogo gomeostaza"* (Proceedings of the third all-Union symposium "The regulation of immune homeostasis"), 113–15. Leningrad.

Shreiber, V. 1963. *The hypothalamo-hypophyseal system.* Prague.

Shtyrova, N. M., and Stankevich, N. V. 1954. Vliyaniye sryva vysshey nervnoy deyatel'nosti na razvitiye difteriynoy intoksikatsii i iskusstvennyy immunitet protiv difterii (The influence of disruption of higher nervous activity on the development of diphtherial intoxication and artificial immunity against diphtheria). In *Problema reaktivnosti v patologii* (The problem of reactivity in pathology), 120–22. Moscow.

Shul'gina, N. S.; Golubeva, N. N.; Korneva, Ye. A.; Pikhtar', V. I.; Savchuk, L. N.; and Marat, B. A. 1973. Osobennosti razvitiya ozhogovogo protsessa v rogovoy obolochke u zhivotnykh s podavlennoy funktsiyey antiteloobrazovaniya (Characteristics of the development of the burn process in the cornea in animals wth inhibited function of antibody formation). In *Oftal'mologiya* (Ophthalmology), 3:103–9. Kiev.

Shul'gina, N. S.; Korneva, Ye. A.; Golubeva, N. N.; Marat, B. A.; Tsvetkova, I. P.; Savchuk, L. N.; Gorchiladze, T. Yu.; Nepomnyashchaya, V. M.; Pikhtar', V. I.; and Vardanyan, I. K. 1975. Neyrogumoral'naya i farmakologicheskaya korrektsiya immunologicheskikh protsessov v rogovoy obolochke (Neurohumoral and pharmacologic correction of immune processes in the cornea). In *Neyrogumoral'naya i farmacologicheskaya korrektsiya immunologicheskikh reaktsiy v eksperimente i klinike.* Tez. dokladov (Neurohumoral and pharmacologic correction of immune processes under experimental and clinical conditions. Proceedings), 75–76. Leningrad.

Shumilina, A. I. 1956. Kharakteristika uslovno-reflektornoy deyatel'nosti sobak pri primenenii aminazina (Characteristics of the conditioned reflex activity of dogs after chlorpromazine administration). *Zhurn. Nevropatol. I Psikhiat.* 56(2):116–20.

Slaunwhite, W. R.; Lockie, G. M.; Bach, N.; and Sandberg, A. A. 1962. Inactivity *in vivo* of transcortin-bound cortisol. *Science* 135:1062–63.

Slonecker, G., and Lim, W. C. 1972. Effects of hydrocortisone on the cells in an acute inflammatory exudate. *Lab. Invest.* 27:123-28.

Slyivic, V. S.; Chark, D. W.; and Warr, G. 1975. Effects of oestrogens and pregnancy on the distribution of sheep erythrocytes and antibody response in mice. *Clin. Exp. Immunol.* 20:179-86.

Smirnov, G. D. 1956. Ritmicheskiye elektricheskiye yavleniya v tsentral'-noy nervnoy sisteme, ikh proiskhozhdeniye i funktsional'noye znacheniye (Rhythmic electrical phenomena in the central nervous system, their origin and functional significance). *Usp. Sovrem. Biol.* 42(6):320-42.

Snell, J. 1960. Relationship of chromium phosphate clearance rates to resistance. 1. The effects of some corticosteroids on blood clearance rates in mice. In *Reticuloendothelial structure and function*, 321-30. New York.

Sollertinskaya, T. N. 1958. Vliyaniye ekstirpatsii verkhnikh sheynykh simpaticheskikh uzlov na reflektornuyu deyatel'nost' kory golovnogo mozga krolikov (The influence of extirpation of the superior cervical sympathetic ganglia on the reflex activity of the cerebral cortex of rabbits. Dissertation). Leningrad.

Solomon, G. F. 1969a. Emotion, stress, the central nervous system and immunity. *Ann. N. Y. Acad. Sci.* 164:335-44.

————. 1969b. Stress and antibody response in rat. *Intern. Arch. Allergy Appl. Immunol.* 35:97-104.

Solomon, G. F.; Allansmith, M.; McClellan, B.; and Amkraut, A. 1969. Immunoglobulins in psychiatric patients. *Arch. Gen. Psychiat.* 20:272-77.

Solomon, G. F.; Amkraut, A. A.; and Kasper, P. 1974. Immunity, emotions and stress. Rev. article. *Ann. Clin. Res.* 6:313-22.

Solov'yeva, V. Ya. 1968. Ob uchastii zadnikh yader gipotalamusa v mekhanizmakh ottorzheniya kozhnykh gomotransplantov (The participation of the posterior hypothalamic nuclei in mechanisms of rejection of skin homotransplants. Dissertation). Saratov.

————. 1969. K uchastiyu zadnikh gipotalamicheskikh yader v mekhanizmakh razvitiya plazmotsitarnoy reaktsii v limfaticheskikh uzlakh pri kozhnoy gomotransplantatsii i eksperimental'nom allergicheskom entsefalomiyelite (The participation of the posterior hypothalamic nuclei in mechanisms of the development of a plasmocytic reaction in the lymph nodes upon skin homotransplantation and experimental allergic encephalomyelitis). In *Patofiziologiya infektsionnogo protsessa i allergii* (Pathophysiology of the infectious process and allergy), 177-97. Saratov.

Solun, Ye. N., and Spirina, D. A. 1967. Ob uchastii yader zadnego gipotalamusa v obrazovanii spetsificheskikh antitel pri eksperimental'nom nevrite (The participation of the posterior hypothalamic nuclei in the formation of specific antibodies in experimental neuritis). In *Patofiziologiya*

infektsionnogo protsessa i allergii (Pathophysiology of the infectious process and allergy), 54(2):171–75. Saratov.

Sorkin, E., and Pierpaoli, W. 1970. Gormony i sposobnost' k immunologicheskomu otvetu (Hormones and the ability for an immune response). In *Sovremennyye problemy immunologii i immunopatologii* (Current problems of immunology and immunopathology), 51–59. Leningrad.

Sosenkov, V. A., and Gorbunova, L. V. 1975. Izmeneniye techeniya nekotorykh immunologicheskikh reaktsiy povyshennoy chuvstvitel'nosti v svyazi s povrezhdeniyem zadnikh yader gipotalamusa (Changes in the course of some immune reactions of raised sensitivity in connection with lesions of the posterior hypothalamic nuclei). In *Neyrogumoral'naya i farmakologicheskaya korrektsiya immunologicheskikh reaktsiy v eksperimente i klinike*. Tez. dokladov (Neurohumoral and pharmacologic correction of immune reactions under experimental and clinical conditions. Proceedings), 60–61. Leningrad.

Spector, N. H. 1981. Neurophysiology, immunophysiology, and neuroimmunomodulation. In *Psychoneuroimmunology*, ed. R. Ader, 449–73. New York: Academic Press.

Speranskiy, A. D. 1935. *Elementy postroyeniya teorii meditsiny* (Structural elements of the theory of medicine). Moscow-Leningrad.

Speranskiy, V. V. 1972. Vliyaniye khorionicheskogo gonadotropina na obshchuyu immunologicheskuyu reaktivnost' obrazovaniya antitel i giperchuvstvitel'nost' nemedlennogo i zamedlennogo tipov u morskikh svinok (The influence of chorionic gonadotrophin on the general immune reactivity of antibody formation and on hypersenstivity of the immediate and retarded types in guinea pigs). *Byull. Eksper. Biol. I Med.* 73(6):61–64.

Speranskiy, V. V., and Muslyumova, S. S. 1974. Vliyaniye khorionicheskogo gonadotropina na vaktsinal'nyy leykotsitoz i transformatsiyu limfotsitov, aktivirovannykh fitogemagglyutininom (The influence of chorionic gonadotrophin on vaccination leukocytosis and the transformation of lymphocytes activated by phytohemagglutinin). In *Voprosy biokhimii i immunologii cheloveka i zhivotnykh* (Problems of human and animal biochemistry and immunology), 120–23. Ufa.

Stark, E. 1972. Regulation of ACTH secretion in stressful conditions. *Acta Med. Acad. Sci. Hung.* 29:77–78.

Stein, M.; Schiari, R. C.; and Luparello, T. J. 1969. The hypothalamus and immune processes. *Ann. N. Y. Acad. Sci.* 164(2):463–72.

Stepanyan, E. D. 1966. Vliyaniye vegetativnykh tsentrov gipotalamusa na immunobiologicheskiye funktsii retikulo-endotelial'noy sistemy v norme i pri patologii (The influence of the vegetative centers of the hypothalamus on the immunobiological functions of the reticuloendothelial system

under normal and pathological conditions). In *Materialy vsesoyuzn. konferentsii probl. fiziol. vegetativoy nervnoy sistemy* (Proceedings of the all-union conference on problems of the physiology of the vegetative nervous system), 147–49. Yerevan.

Stevens, J.; Collesides, C.; and Dongherty, T. E. 1965. Effect of cortisol on the incorporation of thymidine-C^{14} into nuclei acid of lymphatic tissue from adrenalectomized CBA-mice. *Endocrinology* 76:1100–8.

Streng, Ch. B., and Nathan, P. 1973. The immune response in steroid deficient mice. *Immunology* 2:559–65.

Strigin, V. A. 1953. Vliyaniye ugneteniya nervnoy sistemy na infektsiyu i immunitet. Vliyaniye dlitel'nogo uretanovo-veronalovogo sna na prokuktsiyu bryushnotifoznykh agglyutininov pri revaktsinatsii (The influence of inhibition of the nervous system on infection and immunity. The influence of prolonged urethane-veronal sleep on the production of typhoid agglutinins upon revaccination). *Zhurn. Mikrobiol., Epidemiol., Immunobiol.* 24(12):19–21.

Sumarokov, A. A. 1955. Vliyaniye medikamentoznogo sna na fagotsitarnuyu reaktsiyu i kletochnyy sostav eksudata bryushnoy polosti myshey (The influence of drug-induced sleep on the phagocytic reaction and cell composition of the exudate of the abdominal cavity of mice). *Zhurn. Mikrobiol., Epidemiol., Immunobiol.* 26(5):62–63.

Susan, G.; Thrasher, L. L.; Bernardis, T.; and Cohen, S. 1971. The immune response in hypothalamic-lesioned and hypophysectomized rats. *Intern. Arch. Allergy Appl. Immunol.* 41:813–20.

Szabó, T.; Babiczky, L.; Ákoshegyi, I.; Matus, F.; Csaba, G.; Simán, J.; Szilvás, R.; and Jankó, L. 1975. ACTH-nak az ellenanyag termelésére és glucocorticoidnak az immunoglobulin koncentrációra gyakorolt hatása (The effect of ACTH on antibody production and the effect of glucocorticoid on immunoglobulin concentration). *Kísérlet Orvostudomány* 27:64–68.

Szentágothai, J.; Flerkó, B.; Mesh, B.; and Halász, B. 1965. *Gipotalamicheskaya regulyatsiya peredney chasti gipofiza* (Hypothalamic regulation of the anterior lobe of the hypophysis). Budapest.

Szentiványi, A., and Filipp, G. 1958. Anaphylaxis and the nervous system. 2. *Ann. Allergy* 16:143–51.

Szentiványi, A., and Székely, J. 1956. Effect of injury and electrical stimulation of hypothalamus on anaphylactic and histamine shock of the guinea pig: A preliminary report. *Ann. Allergy* 14:259.

Taussig, M. J. 1973. Antigenic competition. In *Current topics in microbiology and immunology*, 127–74. Berlin-Heidelberg, New York.

Ten, H. S. and Paetkau, V. 1974. Biphasic effect of cyclic AMP on an immune response. *Nature* 250:505–7.

Teplov, B. M. 1965. *Tipologicheskiye osobennosti vysshey nervnoy deyatel'-nosti cheloveka* (Typological characteristics of human higher nervous activity), no. 5. Moscow.

Thakur, P. K., and Manchanda, S. K. 1969. Hypothalamic influence on the activity of reticuloendothelial system of cat. *Indian J. Physiol. Pharmacol.* 13:10.

Thatcher, J. S.; Houghton, B. C.; and Ziegler, C. H. 1948. Effect of adrenalectomy and adrenal cortical hormone upon the formation of antibodies. *Endocrinology* 43:440–47.

Thompson, J. S.; Crawford, M. K.; Reilly, R. W.; and Severson, C. D. 1967. The effect of oestrogenic hormones on immune responses in normal and irradiated mice. *J. Immunol.* 98:331–35.

Thrasher, S. G.; Bernardis, L. L.; and Cohen, S. 1971. The immune response in hypothalamic-lesioned and hypophysectomized rats. *Intern. Arch. Allergy Appl. Immunol.* 41:813–20.

Thurstone, I. L. 1953. *Multiple-factor analysis.* Chicago.

Tolkunov, B. R. 1968. Statisticheskiye kharakteristiki fonovoy aktivnosti neyronov (Statistical characteristics of the background activity of neurons). In *Statisticheskaya elektrofiziologiya.* Materialy simpoziuma (Statistical electrophysiology. Proceedings of symposium), 1:134–42. Vilnius.

Tonkikh, A. V. 1965. *Gipotalamo-gipofizarnaya oblast' i regulyatsiya fiziologicheskikh funktsiy organizma* (The hypothalamohypophyseal region and the regulation of physiological functions of the organism). Moscow-Leningrad.

Tormey, P. C.; Fudenkerg, H. H.; and Kamin, R. M. 1967. Effect of prednisolone on synthesis of DNA and RNA by human lymphocytes *in vitro. Nature* 213:281–82.

Trankvilitagin, N. N. Nervnaya regulyatsiya allergicheskikh reaktsiy (Neural regulation of allergic reactions). In *Voprosy immunologii* (Problems of immunology), 54–62. Moscow.

Trufakin, V. A.; Lozovoy, V. P.; Noppe, T. P.; Robinson, M. V.; and Chigir', G. N. 1977. Vliyaniye somatotropnogo gormona na autoimmunnyye reaktsii, indutsirovannyye u myshey raznykh genotipov singennymi progretymi eritrotsitami (The effect of somatotropic hormone on autoimmune responses induced in mice of different genotypes by syngenic heated erythrocytes). *Byull. Eksperim. Biol. I Med.* 83(3):305–8.

Tsvetkova, I. P. 1976. Yadra i polya gipotalamusa krolika (Nuclei and areas of the hypothalamus of rabbits). *Arkh. Anat., Gistol. I Embriol.* 71(11):72–78.

_____. 1977. *Gipotalamus krolika (stereotaksicheskiy i tsitoarkhitektonicheskiy atlas)* (The hypothalamus of the rabbit [stereotaxic and cytoarchitectonic atlas]). Leningrad.

Tsypin, A. B., and Mal'tsev, V. N. 1967. Vliyaniye razdrazheniya gipotalamusa na soderzhaniye normal'nykh antitel v syvorotke krovi (The influence of stimulation of the hypothalamus on the content of normal antibodies in blood serum). *Patol. Fiziol.* 11(5):83–84.

Tul'chinskaya, V. P., and Aplyak, I. V. 1955. Immunobiologicheskiye
reaktsii u laboratornykh zhivotnykh, immunizirovannykh zhivoy brut-
selleznoy vaktsinoy pri razlichnykh sostoyaniyakh nervnoy sistemy (Immunobiological reactions in laboratory animals immunized with living
brucella vaccine at various states of the nervous system). *Zhurn. Mikrobiol., Epidemiol., Immunobiol.* 26(5):56–61.

Tyrey, L., and Nalbandov, A. B. 1972. Influence of anterior hypothalamic
lesions on circulating antibody titers in the rat. *Amer. J. Physiol.*
222:179–85.

Uchitel', I. Ya., and Khasman, E. L. 1968. Vliyaniye veshchestv kataboli-
cheskogo i anabolicheskogo deystviya na obrazovaniye antitel (The influence of substances of catabolic and anabolic effect on the formation of
antibodies). In *Voprosy infektsionnoy patologii i immunologii* (Problems
in infectious pathology and immunology), 4:44–45. Moscow.

——. 1975. Tsentral'nyye i gomeostaticheskiye mekhanizmy regulyatsii
immuniteta (Central and homeostatic mechanisms of the regulation of
immunity). In *Neyrogumoral'naya i farmakologicheskaya korrektsiya
immunologicheskikh reaktsiy v eksperimente i klinike. Tez. dokladov*
(Neurohumoral and pharmacologic correction of immune reactions under experimental and clinical conditions. Proceedings), 65–66. Leningrad.

Uchitel', I. Ya., and Maysyuk, A. P. 1952. Vliyaniye okhranitel'nogo tormozheniya (narkoticheskogo sna) na protsessy infektsii i immuniteta
(The influence of protective inhibition [narcotic sleep] on processes of infection and immunity). *Zhurn. Mikrobiol., Epidemiol., Immunobiol.*
23(2):25–28.

Ukolova, M. A., and Bordyushkov, Yu. N. 1963. Vliyaniye elektricheskogo razdrazheniya gipotalamusa na razvitiye eksperimental'nykh opuk-
holey yaichnika (The influence of electrical stimulation of the hypothalamus on the development of experimental ovarian tumors). *Vopr. Onkol.*
9(10):40–43.

Ukolova, M. A.; Bordyushkov, Yu. N.; and Garkavi, L. Kh. 1962. Vliyaniye razdrazheniya gipotalamusa na rost perevivayemykh sarkom (The influence of stimulation of the hypothalamus on the growth of transplanted sarcomas). *Byull. Eksper. Biol. I Med.* 53(5):111–16.

Ultman, J. E.; Hyman, G. A.; and Calder, B. 1963. The occurrence of lymphoma in patients with long-standing hyperthyroidism. *Blood* 21:282–97.

Unanue, E. R. 1975. The regulation of the immune response by macrophages. In *Mononuclear phagocytosis, immunology, infection and pathology*, 721–38. Oxford.

Ungar, J. M. D. 1955. Enhancement of the antigenic activity of toxoids by sympathomimetic drugs. *Brit. Med. J.* 20:20.

Us, L. A. 1973. Sostoyaniye yader perednego gipotalamusa pri vvedenii antisomatotropnoy syvorotki (The state of the nuclei of the anterior hypothalamus upon administration of antisomatotropic serum). In *Fiziologiya, biokhimiya i patologiya endokrinnoy sistemy* (Physiology, biochemistry, and pathology of the endocrine system), 3:66–68. Kiev.

Uteshev, B. S., and Babichev, V. A. 1974. *Ingibitory biosinteza antitel* (Inhibitors of the biosynthesis of antibodies). Moscow.

Uzonova, A. 1974. Changes of cyclic AMP system during immunization. In *Abstr. commun. ninth meet. Fed. Eur. Biochem. Soc.,* 302. Budapest.

Vakar, M. D. 1968. Vliyaniye adrenalina i atsetilkholina na funktsional'noye sostoyaniye yader gipotalamusa i serdechnoy myshtsy v dinamike nervno-distroficheskogo protsessa (The influence of epinephrine and acetylcholine on the functional state of the nuclei of the hypothalamus and heart muscle in the dynamics of the neurodystrophic process). In *Tr. In-ta Norm. I Pat. Fiziol. AMN SSSR* (Proceedings of the Institute of Normal and Pathological Physiology of the USSR Academy of Medical Sciences), 11:13–15.

Val'dman, A. A. 1958. Vliyaniye farmakologicheskikh veshchestv na provedeniye vozbuzhdeniya po spetsificheskoy i diffuznoy afferentnym sistemam (The effect of drugs on the conduction of excitation over the specific and the diffuse afferent systems). In *Novyye dannyye po farmakologii retikulyarnoy formatsii i simpaticheskoy peredachi* (New data on the pharmacology of the reticular formation and sympathetic transmission), 13–36. Leningrad.

Valuyeva, T. K.; Malyzhev, V. A.; and Davydova, T. I. 1982. Formirovaniye kontaktnoy chuvstvitel'nosti k pikrilkhloridu u myshey v otdalennyye sroki posle timektomii pod vliyaniyem timozina i LSV (The development of long-range contact sensitivity to picryl chloride in mice after thymectomy under the influence of thymosine and LSV). In *Materialy dokladov III vsesoyuznogo simpoziuma "Regulyatsiya immunnogo gomeostaza"* (Proceedings of the third all-union symposium "The regulation of immune homeostasis"), 42–43. Leningrad.

Van-Tan'-an'. 1960. Izmeneniya elektricheskoy aktivnosti kory bol'shikh polushariy i gipotalamusa posle ekstirpatsii verkhnikh i nizhnikh sheynykh simpaticheskikh uzlov u krolikov (Changes in the electric activity of the cerebral cortex and the hypothalamus after extirpation of the upper

and lower cervical sympathetic ganglia in rabbits). *Fiziol. Zhurn. SSSR* 46(8):957–65.

Vartanyan, G. A. 1970. *Vzaimodeystviye vozbuzhdeniya i tormozheniya v neyrone* (The interaction of excitation and inhibition in the neuron). Leningrad.

Vasilevskiy, N. N. 1966. Fonovaya i vyzvannaya impul'snaya aktivnost' neyronov (Background and evoked impulse activity of neurons). In *Mekhanizmy deyatel'nosti tsentral'nogo neyrona* (Mechanisms of the activity of the central neuron), 149–78. Moscow-Leningrad.

————. 1968. *Neyronal'nyye mekhanizmy kory bol'shikh polushariy* (Neuronal mechanisms of the cerebral cortex). Leningrad.

Vasil'yev, L. L., and Lapitskiy, D. A. 1944. O parabioticheskom periode anafilakticheskogo shoka (On the parabiotic period of anaphylactic shock). In *Uch. Zap. LGU. seriya biol. nauk* (Proceedings of the Leningrad State University. Biological science series), 77:114–27.

Vasil'yev, N. V. 1963. *Rol' nervnoy sistemy v protsessakh infektsii i immuniteta* (The role of the nervous system in processes of infection and immunity). Tomsk.

Verzilova, O. V., and Kondrat'yeva, L. N. 1968. Impul'snaya aktivnost' depressornykh struktur gipotalamusa pri reflektornykh reaktsiyakh sosudistoy sistemy (Impulse activity of depressor structures of the hypothalamus during reflex reactions of the vascular system). *Byull. Eksp. Biol. I Med.* 8(66):6–8.

Veselkin, P. N. 1963. *Likhoradka* (Fever). Moscow.

Vessey, S. H. 1964. Effects of grouping on levels of circulating antibodies in mice. In *Proc. Soc. Exp. Biol. Med.*, 115:252–55.

Viernstein, L. J., and Grossman, R. J. 1960. Neural discharge pattern in the transmission of sensory information. In *Information theory: Fourth London symposium*, 252–69. London.

Vogralik, M. V. 1966. Predvaritel'nyye dannyye o techenii nekotorykh tipicheskikh patologicheskikh protsessov v usloviyakh eksperimental'nogo povrezhdeniya vegetativnykh yader perednego i zadnego gipotalamusa (Preliminary data on the course of some typical pathological processes under conditions of experimental damage of the vegetative nuclei of the anterior and posterior hypothalamus). In *Fiziologiya i patofiziologiya gipotalamusa* (Physiology and pathophysiology of the hypothalamus), 216–18. Moscow.

Vogt, M. 1954. The concentration of sympathin in different parts of the central nervous system under normal conditions and after the administration of drugs. *J. Physiol.* 123:451–80.

————. 1959. Catecholamines in brain. *Pharmacol. Rev.* 11:483–89.

Volkova-Borzunina, A. M. 1952. Vozbuzhdeniye i tromozheniye v prot-

sesse immunizatsii loshadey—produtsentov antitoksicheskikh syvorotok (Excitation and inhibition in the process of immunization of horses—producers of antitoxic serums). *Zhurn. Mikrobiol., Epidemiol., Immunobiol.* 10:48–52.

Vvedenskiy, N. Ye. 1952. Sootnosheniye mezhdu ritmicheskimi protsessami i funktsional'noy aktivnost'yu vozbuzhdennogo nervno-myshechnogo apparata (The relation between rhythmic processes and the functional activity of the excited neuromuscular apparatus. In *Poln. sob. soch.* (Complete works), 3:84–93. Leningrad.

Vyazov, O. V., and Khodzhayeva, Sh. Kh. 1973. *Rukovodstvo po immunologii* (Handbook on immunology). Moscow.

Vyazovskaya, R. D. 1960. Vliyaniye razdrazheniya i udaleniya verkhnikh sheynykh simpaticheskikh uzlov na perednyuyu dolyu gipofiza v usloviyakh deystviya aminazina (The influence of stimulation and removal of the superior cervical ganglia on the anterior lobe of the hypophysis under conditions of the effect of chlorpromazine). *Probl. Endokrinol.* 6(2):64–73.

Vygodchikov, G. V. 1952. Nekotoryye voprosy immuniteta v svete ucheniya I. P. Pavlova (Some questions of immunity from the point of view of I. P. Pavlov's concepts). *Zhurn. Mikrobiol., Epidemiol., Immunobiol.* 2:3–13.

Wahl, S. M.; Altman, L. C.; and Rosenstreich, D. L. 1975. Inhibition of *in vitro* lymphokine synthesis by glucocorticosteroids. *J. Immunol.* 115:476–81.

Warner, N. L., and Burnet, I. M. 1961. The influence of testosterone treatment on the development of the bursa of Fabricius in the chick embryo. *Aust. J. Biol. Sci.* 580–87.

Watts, H. G. 1971. The role of cyclic AMP in the immunocompetent cell. *Transplantation* 12:229–31.

Weinstein, J., and Melmon, K. L. 1976. Control of immune response by cAMP and lymphocytes that adhere to histamine columns. *Immunology Communications* 5:401–16.

Weissman, I. L., and Levy, R. 1975. *In vitro* cortisone sensitivity of *in vivo* cortisone-resistant thymocytes. *Isr. J. Med. Sci.* 11:884–88.

Werner, G., and Mountcastle, V. B. 1963. The variability of central neural activity in a sensory system and its implications for the central reflection of sensory events. *Neurophysiology* 26:958.

Weston, W.; Claman, H. N.; and Krueger, C. 1973. Site of action of cortisol in cellular immunity. *J. Immunol.* 110:880–83.

White, A., and Goldstein, A. 1970. Thymosin, a thymus hormone influencing lymphoid cell immunological competence. In *Hormones and the immune response*, 3–24. London.

Wyman, L. C. 1929. Studies on suprarenal insufficiency. 6. Anaphylaxis in suprarenalectomized rats. *Amer. J. Physiol.* 89:356–61.

Yakovleva, M. I. 1959. O deystvii aminazina na sosudistyye i dykhatel'nyye reaktsii u koshek v ontogeneze (The effect of chlorpromazine on vascular and respiratory reactions in cats during ontogenesis). In *Issledovaniya po evolyutsii nervnoy deyatel'nosti* (Investigations on the evolution of nervous activity), 194–99. Leningrad.

———. 1960. O vliyanii gormonov mozgovoy chasti nadpochechnikov na reflektornuyu regulyatsiyu serdechno-sosudistoy sistemy i dykhaniya v ontogeneze (The influence of hormones of the adrenal medulla on the reflex regulation of the cardiovascular system and respiration during ontogenesis. Dissertation). Leningrad.

Yamada, A.; Jensen, M. M.; and Rasmussen, A. F., Jr. 1964. Stress and susceptibility to viral infections. 3. Antibody response and viral retention during avoidance-learning stress. In *Proc. Soc. Exp. Biol. Med.* 116:677–80.

Yarilin, A. A., and Polushkina, E. V. 1975. Analiz deystviya adrenalektomii na kletochnyy sostav i reaktivnost' limfoidnoy tkani myshey (Analysis of the effect of adrenalectomy on the cell composition and the reactivity of the lymphoid tissue in mice). In *Neyrogumoral'naya i farmakologicheskaya korrektsiya immunologicheskikh reaktsiy v eksperimente i klinike. Tez. dokladov* (Neurohumoral and pharmacologic correction of immune reactions under experimental and clinical conditions. Proceedings), 79–80. Leningrad.

Yefimova, N. P., and Kalugina, L. V. 1953. Vliyaniye narkoticheskogo sna i khimicheskikh faktorov nervnogo vozbuzhdeniya na obrazovaniye immuniteta pri difterii (The influence of narcotic sleep and chemical factors of nervous excitation on the development of immunity in diptheria). *Zhurn. Mikrobiol., Epidemiol., Immunobiol.* 24(12):21–28.

Yegorov, A. I. 1966. Vliyaniye razdrazheniya gipotalamusa na vyrabotku antitel (The influence of stimulation of the hypothalamus on the production of antibodies). In *Tez. dokladov III ob'edin. nauch. konferentsii Rostovskogo Med In-ta i Nauchnoissled. In-tov* (Proceedings of the third combined scientific conference of the Rostov Medical Institute and Research Institute), 124–25. Rostov-on-Don.

Yekhneva, T. L. 1975. Vliyaniye gidrokortizona na immunnyy otvet u krys raznogo vozrasta (The influence of hydrocortisone on the immune response in rats of various ages). In *Neyrogumoral'naya i farmakologicheskaya korrektsiya immunologicheskikh reaktsiy v eksperimente i klinike. Tez. dokladov* (Neurohumoral and pharmacologic correction of immune reactions under experimental and clinical conditions. Proceedings), 22. Leningrad.

Yelizarova, K. A. 1954. Izmeneniye funktsional'nogo sostoyaniya vegetativnoy nervnoy sistemy u krolikov v protsesse sensibilizatsii (The change
in the functional state of the vegetative nervous system in rabbits in the
process of sensitization). In *Tezisy dokladov v referaty disk. 14-oy nauchnoy sessii Odesskogo Nauchno-issled. Psikhonevrologich. In-ta* (Proceedings and abstracts of discussions at the fourteenth scientific session
of the Odessa Psychoneurologic Research Institute), 52–53. Odessa.

Yeremina, S. A. 1973. O mekhanizme otritsatel'noy obratnoy svyazi v sisteme gipofiz-kora nadpochechnikov v sostoyanii stressa (On the mechanism of negative feedback in the system hypophysis-adrenal cortex in a
state of stress). In *Fiziologiya, biokhimiya i patologiya endokrinnoy sistemy* (Physiology, biochemistry, and pathology of the endocrine system),
3:24–26. Kiev.

Yeremina, S. A.; Druyan, L. E.; and Minakov, V. I. 1970. Vliyaniye koa-
gulyatsii zadnikh yader gipotalamusa na funktsional'noye sostoyaniye gipotalamo-gipofizarno-adrenalovoy sistemy v dinamike sensibilizatsii i
anafilakticheskogo shoka u sobak (The influence of coagulation of the
posterior nuclei of the hypothalamus on the functional state of the hypothalamohypophyseal-adrenal system in the dynamics of sensitization
and anaphylactic shock in dogs). In *Mekhanizmy nekotorykh patologicheskikh protsessov* (Mechanisms of certain pathological processes),
3:190–97. Rostov-on-Don.

Yudayev, N. A.; Antonichev, A. V.; and Rozen, V. B. 1966. Kontsentrat-
siya 17-oksikortikosteroidov v plazme i svyazyvayushchaya sposobnost'
transkortina (The concentration of 17-oxycorticosteroids in the plasma
and the binding power of transcortin). *Probl. Endokrinol. I Gormono-
terap.* 12(5):72–75.

Yurina, N. A.; Remizova, V. A.; Slyusarchuk, V. P.; and Nechayev, Yu. S.
1975. Vliyaniye kortikosteroidov i estrogenov na kletochnyye sistemy
krovi i soyedinitel'noy tkani, uchastvuyushchiye v immunologicheskikh
reaktsiyakh (The influence of corticosteroids and estrogens on cellular
systems and connective tissue participating in immune reactions). In
*Neyrogumoral'naya i farmakologicheskaya korrektsiya immunologi-
cheskikh reaktsiy v eksperimente i klinike. Tez. dokladov* (Neurohumoral
and pharmacologic correction of immune reactions under experimental
and clinical conditions. Proceedings), 77–79. Leningrad.

Zak, K. P.; Tsarenko, V. I.; Filatova, R. S.; Naumenko, N. I.; Khomenko,
B. M.; Vinnitskaya, M. L.; Lukshina, V. V.; and Shlyakhovenko, V. S.
1975. Vliyaniye gidrokortizona na ul'trastrukturu i vnutrikletochnyy ob-
men leykotsitov krovi i organov leykopoeza immunizirovannykh krolikov (The influence of hydrocortisone on the ultrastructure and intracellular metabolism of blood leukocytes and organs of leukopoiesis of

immunized rabbits). In *Neyrogumoral'naya i farmakologicheskaya korrektsiya immunologichekikh reaktsiy v eksperimente i klinike*. Tez. dokladov (Neurohumoral and pharmacological correction of immune reactions under experimental and clinical conditions. Proceedings), 23–24. Leningrad.

Zaychik, A. Sh. 1971. K mekhanizmam stimulyatsii funktsii shchitovidnoy zhelezy (On the mechanisms of stimulation of the function of the thyroid gland). *Probl. Endokrinol.* 17(4):65–68.

Zborovskiy, A. B., and Chistovskiy, O. B. 1963. K voprosu o roli mezhutochnogo mozga v patogeneze streptokokkovogo giperergicheskogo vospaleniya (On the question of the role of the diencephalon in the pathogenesis of streptococcal hyperergic inflammation). In *Allergiya i autoallergiya*. Materialy konferentsii Baku (Allergy and autoallergy. Proceedings of conference, Baku), 87–89.

————. 1975. K izucheniyu mekhanizmov uchastiya gipotalamusa v immunogeneze pri infektsionno-allergicheskom protsesse (On the study of mechanisms of participation of the hypothalamus in immunogenesis in the infectious-allergic process). In *Neyrogumoral'naya i farmakologicheskaya korrektsiya immunologicheskikh reaktsiy v eksperimente i klinike*. Tez. dokladov (Neurohumoral and pharmacologic correction of immune reactions under experimental and clinical conditions. Proceedings), 24–25. Leningrad.

Zdrodovskiy, P. F. 1962. Tsitofiziologicheskiye mekhanizmy immunogeneza (Cytophysiological mechanisms of immunogenesis). *Vestn. AMN SSSR* 17(4):57–65.

————. 1969. *Problemy infektsii, immuniteta i allergii* (Problems of infection, immunity, and allergy). Moscow.

————. 1971. O fiziologicheskikh aspektakh immunogeneza i yego regulyatsii (On physiological aspects of immunogenesis and its regulation). *Vestn. AMN SSSR* 26(12):41–48.

Zdrodovskiy, P. F., and Gurvich, G. A. 1972. *Fiziologicheskiye osnovy immunogeneza i yego regulyatsii* (Physiological principles of immunogenesis and its regulation). Moscow.

Zdrodovskiy, P. F.; Gurvich, G. A.; and Kabanova, Ye. A. 1973. O fiziologicheskikh aspektakh immunogeneza i yego regulyatsii (On physiological aspects of immunogenesis and its regulation). *Zhurn. Gigiyeny, Epidemiol., Mikrobiol., Immunol.* 17(1):34–44.

Zelenskaya, V. S., and Pyatigorskiy, B. Ya. 1968. Fonovaya aktivnost' neyronov blednogo shara (Background activity of the neurons of the globus pallidus). In *Statisticheskaya elektrofiziologiya* (Statistical electrophysiology), 2:217–24. Vilnius.

Zenzerov, V. S.; Dedov, I. I.; and Yakovlev, V. A. 1973. Shchitovidnaya zheleza v usloviyakh kholodnvogo stressa (The thyroid gland in conditions of cold stress). In *Stress i yego patogeneticheskiye mekhanizmy* (Stress and its pathogenetic mechanisms), 207–8. Kishinev.

Zhukova, S. V. 1960. Vliyaniye razdrazheniya verkhnikh sheynykh simpaticheskikh uzlov na nervnyye kletki supraopticheskogo yadra (The influence of stimulation of the superior cervical sympathetic ganglia on the nerve cells of the supraoptic nucleus). In *Tezisy dokladov 1-oy konferentsii morfologov-endokrinologov* (Proceedings of the first conference of morphologists-endocrinologists), 35–36. Leningrad.

Zil'ber, L. A. 1958. *Osnovy immunologii* (Principles of immunology). Moscow.

Znachkova, A. A. 1945. Vliyaniye nervnoy sistemy na vyrabotku antitel (The influence of the nervous system on the production of antibodies. Dissertation). Moscow.

Zotova, V. V. 1967. K voprosu o roli gipotalamicheskoy oblasti v protsesse immunogeneza (On the role of the hypothalamic region in the process of immunogenesis). In *Mekhanizmy nekotorykh patologicheskikh protsessov* (Mechanisms of certain pathological processes), 1:13–22. Rostov-on-Don.

————. 1968. K voprosu o roli gipotalamicheskoy oblasti v formirovanii nekotorykh immunologicheskikh reaktsiy (On the role of the hypothalamic region in the development of certain immune reactions. Dissertation). Donetsk.

Zubzhitskiy, Yu. N., and Ogurtsov, R. P. 1976. Nekotoryye voprosy prikladnogo ispol'zovaniya fenomena immunologicheskoy pamyati (Some questions of applied utilization of the phenomenon of immunologic memory). In *Pamyat' v mekhanizmakh normal'nykh i patologicheskikh reaktsiy* (Memory in mechanisms of normal and pathological reactions), 253–69. Leningrad.

Author Index

Abavari, K., 3, 123, 126, 166
Abinder, A. A., 45
Ablin, R. F., 144
Ach, Zs., 3, 123, 125
Adam, J., 88
Adamov, A. K., 147
Adler, F. L., 96
Adner, M. M., 144
Ado, A. D., 9, 10, 11, 15, 17, 38, 39, 51
Aikawa, S., 59
Akimova, R. N., 31
Akoshegyi, I., 100
Aleshin, B. V., 17, 30, 112, 116, 127, 132, 152
Alexander, P., 147
Alifanov, V. V., 64
Alperina, Ye. L., 171
Al'pern, D., 51, 137
Altman, L. C., 105
Ambrose, C. T., 100, 101, 102, 141
Amkraut, A. A., 38
Anand, B. K., 58
Andersen, P., 64
Andersson, B., 106, 107
Anokhin, P. K., 18, 23
Antonichev, A. V., 125

Aplyak, I. V., 6
Arutyunyan, V. M., 148
Ass-Babich, B. T., 148
Astaf'yeva, N. G., 33
Astrauskas, V. I., 51, 137, 158
Asyamolova, I. A., 23
Aver'yanova, L. L., 17
Avetikyan, B., 15
Azhipa, Ya. I., 18, 24
Aznauryan, A. V., 148

Babichev, V. A., 104, 105
Babiczky, L., 100
Bach, J. F., 107
Bach, N., 123
Baguena, J., 101
Baguena, R., 101
Baklavadzhan, O. G., 30
Balabolkin, M. I., 147
Balow, J. E., 103, 104
Bardakhch'yan, E. A., 38
Baroni, C., 118, 149
Barraclough, C. A., 58
Bartter, F. P., 125
Baust, W., 58
Baydakov, P. A., 11
Beck, N. P., 110

Bedretdinov, Kh. A., 73
Bekhtereva, N. P., 73, 169
Belasic, M., 16
Belbey, D. L. J., 105
Belenev, Yu., 108, 122, 123, 125
Belen'kiy, G. S., 8
Beling, C. C., 144
Belovolova, R. A., 120, 122, 139, 141
Belyavskiy, A. D., 6, 10, 122
Benetato, Gr., 32, 33, 118
Bennett, M., 105
Berger, M., 23
Berglund, K., 100, 101, 102
Beritov, I. S., 56
Bernardis, L. L., 38, 118
Bernasconi, C., 105
Bernett, F., 1, 96, 103
Bielski, R. K., 144
Bilenko, V. I., 103
Biryukov, D. A., 3, 23
Blomgren, H., 106, 107
Bogdanchikova, V. V., 33, 38
Bogendorfer, L., 7
Bondarev, I. M., 56
Bonvallet, M., 18
Bordyushkov, Yu. N., 45
Botkin, S. P., vii, viii
Bosing-Scheider, R., 110
Braun, W., 110
Brighenti, L., 101
Brooks, C. M. C., 55
Broun, G. R., 56, 58
Brown, G. M., 116
Budylin, N. V., 6
Bullock, T. H., 57
Bundzen, P. V., 73
Burnett, I. M., 144
Burns, B. D., 63
Burykina, G. N., 51
Buss, H., 88
Buss, K., 88

Cabanac, M., 58
Calder, B., 148
Cannon, W. B., 24
Castro, J. E., 144
Chang, S., 115
Chaplinskiy, V. Ya., 148
Char, D. F. B., 117
Chebotarev, V. R., 100, 104, 118
Chen, H. J., 116
Chen, H. T., 116
Chen, P. S., 125
Cherednichenko, R. P., 24, 53
Chernigovskaya, N. V., 51
Chernukh, A. M., 16, 159, 161
Cherry, C. P., 144
Chertkov, I. L., 103
Chigir', G. N., 170
Chistovskiy, O. B., 45, 51
Chtetsov, V. P., 73
Chubukhchiyev, V. Kh., 167
Church, A. B., 105
Claman, H. N., 105, 106, 110
Code, C. F., 118, 137
Cohen, E. P., 107
Cohen, J. J., 107, 168
Cohen, P., 107
Cohen, S., 38, 118
Cole, L. L., 105
Collesides, C., 109
Comstock, J. P., 108
Coons, A. H., 101
Cooper, S., 103
Corson, E. O'L., ix
Corson, S. A., viii
Cox, D. R., 65, 66, 70, 80
Craddock, C. S., 104, 105
Crawford, M. K., 144
Criep, L. H., 117
Cross, B. A., 30, 57, 58, 61
Csaba, G., 100
Cudkowich, Z. L., 105

Dafny, N., 30, 58, 60
Dameshen, W., 144
Danilova, O. A., 128
Dannenberg, A., 105
Danute, J. S., 110
Dardenne, M., 107
Darrach, M., 100, 101, 102, 111
Darzynkiewicz, Z. 103
Daughaday, W. H., 125
Deckx, R., 123
Dedov, I. I., 116
Delespesse, G., 168
Denef, C., 123
Denisenko, P. P., 24, 53, 137
Dertouzos, M., 67
Devoyno, L. V., 50, 53, 141, 171
Dews, P. B., 118, 137
Dias, S. W., 110
Dibbot, J. A., 116
Dietrich, F. M., 100, 102
Doe, R. P., 123
Dolin, A. O., 8, 9
Dongherty, T. E., 109
Dougherty, T. F., 103, 104, 105, 106
Ducor, P., 100, 102
Dugueskoy, R. J., 110, 118, 149
Dunn, J. D., 116
D'yachenko, S. S., 100, 101

Eastman, C. J., 101, 116
Ebert, L. Ya., 15
Eccles, J. C., 64
Ehrlich, P., vii
Eisenman, J. S., 57
Eisenstein, A., 107
Eives, M. W., 103
Endröczi, E., 112, 127, 132, 152
Enenkel, H. J., 15
Engelhardt, G., 24
Enke, H., 88
Ernstrom, U., 148
Eskin, I. A., 152

Esteban, J. N., 105
Evans, M. M., 118
Everett, J. W., 33
Eylan, E., 147

Fabris, N., 147, 148, 149
Fagraens, A., 100, 102
Fanci, A. S., 106
Fedorov, Yu. V., 6
Fedoseyev, G. V., 171
Fedotov, V. P., 117
Feldman, S., 30, 58, 60
Felsenfeld, O., 114
Fenichel, G., 32
Fernandes, G., 116
Fialkow, P., 105
Fifkova, E., 33, 63
Filimonov, V. G., 56
Filipp, G., 31, 38, 39, 134, 137
Findlay, A. L. R., 60
Fintiktinova, R. P., 6
Firsova, P. P., 6
Fischel, E. E., 101, 102
Flerov, B. A., 9
Franchimont, P., 116
Freedman, D. X., 32
Freundt, G. P., 110
Fridenshteyn, A., Ya., 103
Frolov, Ye. P., 10, 14, 16, 25, 39, 45,
    117, 141
Fryazinova, I. B., 105
Fudenkerg, H. H., 103, 104
Fujii, H., 144

Gabourei, J. D., 109
Gamaleya, N. F., 14
Ganenko, D. M., 73
Garkavi, L. Kh., 45
Garvey, J. S., 101, 102
Gaumer, H. R., 105
Gavin, J., 147
Gavrilova, L. N., 18

Gavrilova, T. M., 38
Gellhorn, E., 24
Genkin, A. A., 126
Germanov, N. I., 6
Gershon, R. C., 107
Gerstein, G. L., 59, 64, 65
Gioelli, A., 101
Gisler, R. H., 114, 152
Glazyrina, P. V., 11
Glezer, V. D., 57, 63
Glick, B., 144, 147
Gogolitsin, Yu. L., 73
Gol'dshteyn, M. M., 38
Goldstein, A., 101
Golikov, N. V., 56
Golovkova, I. N., 8
Golubeva, N. N., 25, 39, 47, 49, 51,
    53, 171
Good, R. A., 110
Gorbunova, L. V., 40
Gordiyenko, A. N., 9, 10, 16, 24,
    25, 56
Gordon, D. S., 171
Gordon, M. A., 168
Goreen, P., 147
Grachev, G. I., 56
Granit, R., 57
Grashchenkov, N. I., 52
Green, G. D., 55, 57
Green, J. D., 33
Greer, W. E., 114
Grigor'yev, V. A., 170
Gromova, Ye. A., 55
Groot, J. de, 40
Grossman, R. G., 64
Gubler, Ye. V., 126
Gul'yants, E. S., 38
Gurvich, G. A., 31, 100, 104, 114,
    115, 118, 145, 146, 147
Gushchin, G. V., 53
Gushchin, I. S., 39, 51
Gutorova, N. M., 120

Hadden, E. M., 25, 168
Hadden, J. W., 25, 168
Hagiwara, S., 59
Halliday, W. J., 101, 102
Hammond, C. W., 101
Han, T., 144
Hanai, T., 57
Hanjan, S. N. S., 147
Hansen, H. G., 103
Haolden, J. W., 110
Hardy, J. D., 57
Harris, G., 40
Havlicek, V., 58
Hayashida, T., 100, 146
Hayward, J. N., 60
Hejco, E., 116
Hessalsjo, R., 146
Heuser, G., 146
Hilgar, A. G., 104
Hill, C. W., 114
Hirsch, J. G., 105
Holm, E., 73
Holne, R., 146
Houghton, B. C., 118, 137
Huang, J. Ch., 110
Hunt, C. C., 57
Hyman, G. A., 148

Illner, P., 116
Ingle, D. I., 141
Ioffe, V. I., 3, 4, 75, 120
Irvine, W. J., 118
Isakovic, K., 38, 39
Ishidate, J., 103
Ishimova, L. M., 9, 10, 39, 56
Ishizuka, M., 25, 110
Ivanov, V. M., 101, 118
Ivanus, J., 39
Izotov, V. K., 146

Janko, L., 100
Jankovic, B. D., 38, 39

Jones, M. A., 103
Jones, W., 144
Jong, W., 110

Kabanova, Ye. A., 145
Kakhana, M. S., 52
Kalden, Y. R., 118
Kalugina, L. V., 15
Kamin, R. M., 103, 104
Kanarevskaya, A. A ., 31
Kanda, R., 39
Kaplunovskiy, A. S., 73, 75
Karady, S., 8
Karamyan, A. I., 18, 22
Karmali, R. A., 144
Karpov, M. K., 6
Kass, E., 158
Katani, M., 144
Katz, P., 58
Kavetsky, R. E., 31
Kaye, M., 144
Kaznacheyev, V. P., 1
Kebadze, N. N., 148
Kelley, V. C., 117
Kemp, R. G., 110
Khasman, E. L., 51, 100
Khay, L. M., 3, 4, 17, 21, 33, 40, 42,
    43, 47, 50, 82, 83, 169
Khayetsky, J. K., 31
Khlebutina, T. A., 40
Khodzhayeva, Sh. Kh., 120
Khoruzhaya, T. A., 137, 138
Khozak, L. Ye., 11
Kiang, N. Y. S., 59, 64, 65
Kibyakov, A. V., 21
Kinnaert, P., 105
Kiseleva, V. I., 56
Kishkovskaya, O. V., 48, 49
Kiss, L., 8
Kitay, G. J., 30
Klegg, A., 111
Klegg, P., 111

Klimenko, V. M., 59, 67, 73, 75, 170
Knigge, K. M., 131
Kogan, A. B., 16, 57, 70, 83
Komissarenko, V. P., 111, 112, 157
Konar, D. B., 38, 47
Kondrat'yeva, L. N., 58
Konovalov, G. V., 51
Kopytovskaya, L. P., 21, 100, 117
Korneva, E. A., 17, 21, 33, 40, 42,
    43, 48, 50, 52, 59, 82, 83, 168,
    169, 170
Kostinskiy, D. D., 144
Kostyuk, P. G., 57, 60
Kovacs, A., 39
Kovaleva, I. G., 146
Koyi, S., 57
Kozlov, V. A., 170
Kozlov, V. K., 14, 16, 17, 53, 104,
    107, 117, 141
Kraskina, N. A., 120
Krueger, C., 106
Krulich, L., 116
Krylov, S. S., 51
Krylov, V. N., 8, 9
Kulikov, M. A., 64, 65
Kuno, M., 57
Kurashvili, V. Ye., 6, 7, 15, 16
Kuznetsov, S. M., 9

Laborit, H., 159
Ladosz, J., 25
Laguchev, S. S., 103
Lance, E. M., 103
Lapitskiy, D. A., 6
Larson, B., 148
Larson, D., 101
Lavender, J. F., 115
Lazar, L., 39
Lazarev, A. F., 146
Lebedev, A. N., 56, 57
Lee, K., 153
Lendle, L., 24

Leonavichene, L. K., 51, 137, 170
Lesniak, M., 147
Levick, W. R., 64
Levine, M. A., 106
Levy, R., 107
Lewis, P. A., 65, 66, 70, 80
Leytes, S. M., 141
Li, C. H., 100, 146
Lim, W. C., 105
Lissak, K., 112, 127, 132, 152
Litvak, R. V., 15
Livanov, M. N., 56, 57, 61
Lockie, G. M., 123
London, Ye. S., 5, 7
Long, D. A., 105
Lowry, O. H., 123
Lozovoy, V. P., 170
Lukicheva, T. I., 16, 45
Luk'yanenko, V. I., 9
Lundin, P. M., 52, 118, 146
Luparello, T. J., 38, 51
Luria, M. V., 105
Lutskiy, V. A., 56, 57

McIntyre, H. B., 116
MacManus, J. P., 25
Maestroni, G. J. M., 168
Maginskis, V. A., 59, 64
Mahieu, A., 105
Makara, G. B., 30, 127
Makarenko, Yu. A., 25
Mallyrek, J., 146
Malt'sev, V. N., 40, 41
Mamikonyan, R. S., 148
Manchanda, S. K., 38, 47
Maor, D., 147
Marakusha, I. G., 50
Marat, B. A., 46, 47, 49, 50, 117
March, J. T., 115
Marchuk, P. D., 15
Markov, Kh. M., 56
Maros, T., 39

Marschal, D., 33, 63
Maruyama, N., 57
Mashkovskiy, M. D., 23
Mats-Rossinskaya, V. S., 6
Matus, F., 100
Matveichuck, Y. D., 31
Maysyuk, A. P., 6
Mechnikov, I. I., vii, ix
Mednieks, M. I., 110
Medvedev, V. M., 17
Medvedeva, M. V., 3
Meites, J., 116
Melikhova, M. A., 61
Melkumyan, M. A., 15
Melmon, K. L., 168
Mel'nikov, V. N., 6, 15
Menitskiy, D. N., 57
Meshalova, A. N., 100, 101, 102, 105
Mess, B., 32, 134, 137
Metal'nikov, A., 168
Metcalf, D., 103, 105
Middleton, E., 25, 168
Mihaly, K., 30, 127
Mikaelyan, M. G., 148
Mikhaylov, V. V., 33, 40, 50
Mikhaylova, N. V., 104, 168
Miller, J. F., 103, 105, 153
Mills, J. H., 125
Mirick, G. S., 101
Mitel'man, P. M., 6
Mody, E., 39
Moeschlin, S., 101
Moiseyeva, N. I., 3
Moll, J. de, 116
Molomut, N., 118
Monayenkov, A. M., 7, 8
Moor, P. de, 123
Moore, G. P., 64
Morenkov, E. S., 40
Morgunov, I. N., 15
Morin, F., 55

Mountcastle, V. B., 57, 65
Mueller, G. P., 116
Murphy, J. T., 58
Muslyumova, S. S., 144
Mustardy, L., 8

Nakayama, H., 59
Nakayama, T., 57
Nalbandov, A. B., 118, 134
Narushevichus, J. B., 59, 64
Nasonov, D. N., 56
Nathan, P., 117
Nauta, J. H., 36
Nauta, W. J., 39, 131
Nawa, G., 144
Nebylitsyn, V. D., 71, 73
Nechayev, Yu. S., 104, 144
Nesterenko, K. A., 6
Newson, S. E., 100
Nicol, T., 105
Nikolayev, N. I., 147
Nishioka, S., 59
Noppe, T. P., 170
Northe, R., 105
Novak, M., 101

Odell, W. D., 116
Ogurtsov, R. P., 39, 48, 50
Oleynikova, Ye. A., 6
Oliveira, L. A., 110
Orlova, L. N., 6
Otsuka, T., 59
Overall, J. E., 88
Oyvin, I. A., 10

Paetkau, V., 110
Palant, B. L., 6
Palkovits, M., 30, 127
Pankov, Yu. A., 120
Pankova, S. S., 125
Park, B. H., 110
Park, C. D., 51

Paulsen, F., 146
Pavlov, I. P., vii
Pedal, H. W., 15
Pel'ts, D. G., 8, 116
Penneman, R., 105
Perelygina, T. M., 33
Perkel, D. H., 57, 64
Petrov, R. V., 1, 13, 36, 46, 96, 103, 104, 118, 168
Petrovskiy, I. N., 40
Pienkowski, M., 103
Pierpaoli, W., 118, 145, 147, 149, 168
Pillai, P. V., 58
Plescia, O. J., 110
Pletsityy, D. F., 7
Plokhinskiy, N. A., 67, 162
Podpolzin, A. A., 24, 38
Poggio, G. F., 57, 59
Polenov, A. L., 30
Polishchuk, I. A., 23
Poltavchenko, G. M., 168
Polushkin, B. V., 16
Polushkina, E. V., 117
Polyak, A. I., 33, 48, 50, 51, 139, 141, 170
Ponomarev, A. V., 15
Popjak, G., 17
Poth, J., 147
Potin, V. V., 52
Povazhenko, A. A., 116
Powell, T. P., 57
Preobrazhenskiy, N. I., 59
Pronin, L. A., 7
Pyatigorskiy, B. Ya., 59
Pytskaya, Ye. G., 138
Pytskiy, V. I., 17, 138

Queiroz, J. M., 110

Rabina, E. V., 51
Rafika, M. O., 11

Rasmussen, A. F., 115
Raus, J., 123
Read, C. B., 116
Reichlin, S., 116
Reilly, R. W., 144
Remizova, V. A., 104, 144
Renaud, L. P., 58
Repin, I. S., 10
Revesz, T., 30, 127
Reznikov, A. G., 111, 112, 157
Riudani, T. H., 146
Roberts, S., 118
Robinson, M. V., 170
Rodieck, R. W., 64, 65
Rodshteyn, O. A., 51
Rose, B., 102, 105, 137
Rosenstreich, D. L., 105
Rozen, V. B., 108, 122, 123, 125
Rozental', K. M., 75, 120
Ruben, L. N., 100
Rumbesht, L. M., 33, 48, 51
Ryzhenkov, V. Ye., 128

Saakov, B. A., 33, 38
Sakanyan, S. Sh., 148
Sandberg, A. A., 123
Savchenko, I. G., 5, 7, 168
Savchuk, O. Ye., 8, 71
Sawa, M., 57
Sawyer, C. H., 33
Schaefer, H., 73
Schedl, H. P., 125
Schellin, U., 146
Schenkel-Hullinger, L., 114
Schmutzler, W., 110
Schneebeli, G. L., 103, 105
Schulman, J. H., 57
Schwarz, M. R., 144
Schwell, S., 105
Seal, U. S., 123
Sechenov, I. M., vii, ix
Segundo, J. P., 57, 64

Selye, H., 100, 113, 115, 116
Sergeyev, G. A., 64
Sergeyev, P. V., 100, 101, 102, 107, 109, 113
Sergeyev, Yu. V., 10
Sergeyeva, V. Ye., 171
Serov, V. V., 51
Severson, C. D., 144
Shakharova, G. G., 50
Shakhbazyan, P. T., 148
Shannon, A. D., 103
Shapiro, A. I., 100
Shapovalov, A. I., 57
Shargin, S. M., 116
Shatilova, N. V., 16, 45
Shekoyan, V. A., 47, 51, 170
Shemerovskaya, T. G., 101, 102, 144, 146
Shepotinovskiy, V. I., 40
Sherman, J. D., 144
Shimamura, T., 110
Shkhinek, E. K., 51, 120, 123, 126, 127, 131, 132, 134, 166, 168, 170
Shreiber, V., 116, 127, 152
Shtokolova, R. A., 51
Shtyrova, N. M., 7
Shul'gina, G. I., 39, 47, 49, 61
Shumilina, A. I., 23
Silver, I. A., 58, 61
Siman, J., 100
Sklenovsky, A., 58
Skott, D. E., 131
Slaunwhite, W. R., 123
Sloneker, G., 105
Slyusarchuk, V. P., 104, 144
Slyvic, V. S., 144
Smirnov, G. D., 56
Snell, J., 105
Sokolov, A. Ya., 117
Sollertinskaya, T. N., 18, 20, 21, 22
Solomon, G. F., 38, 50, 113, 114
Solov'yeva, V. Ya., 33, 40, 50

Sorkin, E., 118, 145, 147, 149
Spector, N., ix
Speranskiy, A. D., 31, 168
Speranskiy, V. V., 143
Stankevich, N. V., 7
Stark, E., 30, 127
Stein, M., 38, 51
Stepanyan, E. D., 41
Stepanyan, M. S., 148
Stepushkina, T. A., 56
Stevens, J., 109
Streng, Ch. B., 117
Strokova, I. G., 122, 125
Subbotin, M. Ya., 1
Sudakov, K. V., 24
Sumarokov, A. A., 6
Swartz, I., 105
Szabo, T., 100
Szalai, K., 3, 126, 166
Szekely, J., 40
Szentagothai, J., 31, 36, 127
Szentivanyi, A., 32, 40
Szilvas, R., 100

Talwar, G. P., 147
Taussig, M. J., 131
Ten, H. S., 110
Teplov, B. M., 73
Tevosyan, E. Ye., 148
Thatcher, J. S., 118, 137
Thompson, J. S., 144
Thrasher, S. G., 38, 118
Thurstone, I. L., 73
Tolkunov, B. R., 58, 59, 65, 70
Tolmacheva, N. S., 16
Tomlinson, L., 101
Tonkikh, A. V., 30
Tormey, P. C., 103, 104
Torosyan, S. Ye., 148
Trankvilitagin, N. N., 16
Trufakin, V. A., 170
Tsvetkova, I. P., 3, 28, 29, 33, 36

Tsypin, A. B., 40, 41
Tsyrlova, I. G., 104
Tul'chinskaya, V. P., 6
Turkevich, N. M., 31
Tyrey, L., 118, 134

Uchitel', I. Ya., 6, 100
Ukolova, M. A., 45
Ultman, J. E., 148
Unanue, E. R., 103, 153
Undritsov, M. I., 16, 45
Ungar, J. M. D., 15
Usvatova, I. Ya., 120
Uteshev, B. S., 104, 105
Uzonova, A., 110

Vakar, M. D., 15
Val'dman, A. A., 23
Valuyeva, T. K., 118, 170
Van-Tan'-an', 18, 20, 22
Vartanyan, G. A., 57
Vasguez, P. L., 110
Vashetko, V. A., 23
Vasilevskiy, N. N., 56, 57, 59, 60, 61, 65, 70
Vasil'yev, L. L., 6, 9, 25
Vaughan, M. R., 100
Verzilova, O. V., 58
Veselkin, P. N., 4, 10
Vessey, S. H., 114
Viernstein, L. F., 59, 64
Vilkov, G. A., 138
Vinitskaya, Ye. B., 16, 45
Vogralik, M. V., 51
Vogt, M., 24
Volchek, A. G., 108, 122, 123, 125
Volkova-Borzunina, A. M., 7
Vvedinskiy, N. Ye., 56
Vyazov, O. V., 120
Vyazovskaya, R. D., 18
Vygodchikov, G. V., 7

Wahl, S. M., 105
Warner, N. L., 144
Watts, H. G., 25
Weinstein, J., 168
Weissman, I. L., 107
Weksler, M. E., 144
Werner, G., 65
Weston, W., 106
White, A., 101, 103, 118
Whitfield, J. F., 25
Williams, C. M., 88
Williams, W. C., 64
Wilson, I. B., 168
Wyman, L. C., 21

Yakovlev, V. A., 116
Yakovleva, M. I., 21, 23
Yamada, A., 113
Yamamoto, I., 110
Yarilin, A. A., 117
Yarovitskiy, N. V., 59
Yefimova, N. P., 15
Yegorov, A. I., 40
Yekhneva, T. L., 100, 104

Yelizarova, K. A., 15
Yeremina, S. A., 53, 137
Yondale, T., 25
Yudayev, N. A., 125
Yurina, N. A., 104, 144

Zak, K. P., 103, 106
Zakharchenko, Ye. P., 33
Zappazodi, P., 105
Zaretskaya, Yu. M., 96
Zaychik, A. Sh., 116
Zborovskiy, A. B., 45, 51
Zdrodovskiy, P. F., 6, 9, 31, 98, 100,
    101, 104, 114, 115, 118, 145, 146,
    147
Zelenskaya, V. S., 59
Zenzerov, V. S., 116
Zhabotinskiy, Yu. M., 4
Zhukova, S. V., 18
Ziegler, C. H., 118, 137
Zil'ber, L. A., 9
Znachkova, A. A., 17
Zotova, V. V., 33, 48, 50, 51
Zubzhitskiy, Yu, N., 4, 39, 48, 50

Subject Index

ACTH, effects on immune
reactions, 103–5, 140
Adrenalectomy, effects on immune
reactions, 117
Adrenaline, effects on blood levels
of antibodies, 15
Adrenal medulla
demedullation, 21, 22
immune reactions, 21, 22
Adrenergic system, activation of
immune reactions, 53
Allergic reactions and
glucocorticoids, 138
Alpha-adrenergic blocking drugs
and immunoblocking effects,
171
Amphetamine, intensification of
immune reactions, 6, 15, 171
Amygdala and immune reactions,
170
Anaphylaxis and hypothalamus,
137
Androgens and immune reactions,
144
Antigen entry into organism
effects on excitation in amygdala,
170
effects on hormonal shifts, 156,

170
effects on posterior
hypothalamus, 170
effects on sympathoadrenal
system, 27
glucocorticoid release as
nonspecific reaction to
stressors, 165
release of mineralocorticoids, 170
Arthus phenomenon, 137
Autonomic nervous system and
immune reactions, 14

B-lymphocytes, 13
Bursa of Fabricius and bone stem
cells, 13

Caffeine, intensification of immune
reactions, 6
Catecholamines
activation of cell division of
thymocytes and lymphoid
cells, 27
increase during early stages of
immunogenesis, 25
intensification of activity of
adenylcyclase in lymphoid
tissue cells, 25

stimulation of phagocytes, 25
Cervical sympathetic nerve
    transection and immune
    reactions, 16
Chlorpromazine and immune
    reactions, 23
Cholinergic system and immune
    reactions, 53
Chorionic gonadotropins and
    immune reactions, 144
CNS lesions
    inhibition of immune reactions, 7
    suppression of antibody
        formation, 7
CNS stimulants, intensification of
    immune reactions, 6
Cold stress, effects on plasmocyte
    reactions, 115
Conditioned reflexes
    anaphylactic reaction, 9
    intensity of antibody formation,
        7, 8, 9, 11
    mobilization of antibodies, 8
    production of antibodies, 8

Dexamethasone, effects on immune
    reactions, 132, 135
Diurnal rhythms of hormones and
    immune reactions, 116

Emotions and immune reactions, 31
Endocrines
    effects of hypophysio-
        adrenocortical system, 99, 113,
        114
    effects on immune reactions, 98
    mechanisms of action, 109, 110,
        111, 139, 140, 141
Endogenous hormones, effects on
    immune reactions, 113-39
    corticosteroids, 142
    hormones of the hypophysio-

adrenocortical system, 113,
    142
Estrogens and immune reactions,
    144
Exogenous hormones, effects on
    immune reactions, 100, 101
    ACTH, 103, 110
    glucocorticoids, 102, 105, 107,
        108

Glucocorticoids, effects on immune
    reactions, 102-8
    mechanism of effects, 109, 110,
        120, 152, 153, 154, 165
Growth hormone and immune
    reactions, 146

Hippocampus and immune
    reactions, 170
Humoral factors of bone marrow,
    168
Hypophysio-adrenocortical system,
    effects of exogenous
    hormones, 100, 101
Hypophysectomy, effects on
    immune reactions, 118
Hypothalamic neurons
    activity in immune reactions, 80-
        97
    baseline electrical activity and
        functional state, 56, 57, 58
    factor analysis of neuronal
        impulsation during
        immunogenesis, 96, 97
    frequency of neuronal impulses,
        62, 63
    histograms of impulse intervals,
        64-73
    quantitative characterization of
        neuronal impulse activity
        during immunogenesis, 59-83,
        88

Hypothalamus and immune
    reactions, 29, 55
  effects on antigen-antibody
    reactions, 32
  effects of stimulation on
    dynamics of tumor
    development, 45
  effects of stimulation on immune
    reactions, 40
  effects on cellular immunity, 40,
    50
  influence on inductive phase of
    immunization and on antigen
    elimination, 47
  integrative functions, 30
  intensity of phagocytic reaction,
    33
  lesions in, and maturation of
    lymphoid cells, 46
  nonspecific resistance, 32
Hypothalamus, anterior, 45
  effects of stimulation on immune
    reactions, 45
Hypothalamus, medial
  electrocoagulation, 32
  inhibition of anaphylactic shock,
    32
Hypothalamus, posterior
  antibody production, 33, 34
  antigen elimination, 33, 34
  damage and hypertrophy of
    endothelial cells, 36
  damage and hypertrophy of glial
    elements, 36
  effects of stimulation and
    location of electrodes, 44
  immune reactions, 33, 34, 38
  lesions in and decrease in
    macrophage lysosomal activity,
    46, 47
  lesions in and decrease in number
    of antibody-producing cells,

    33, 48
  lesions in and decrease in number
    of sensitized lymphocytes in
    spleen and lymph nodes, 47, 48
  lesions in and decrease in plasma
    concentrations of 11–OH–CS,
    128, 129
  lesions in and hyperplasia and
    hypertrophy of glial elements,
    36
  lesions in and prolongation of
    survival of homotransplanted
    skin flaps, 50
  stimulation of and antibody
    production, 44

Immune reactions
  to brucellosis allergies, 6
  to dysentery bacillus, 6
  genetic differences, 9
  involvement of neural and
    humoral pathways, 164, 165
  to pertussis vaccine, 6
  to tick-borne encephalitis virus, 6
  to typhoid vaccine, 6
Immunization
  increased excitability in the
    amygdala, 170
  increases in total plasma 11–OH–
    CS, inductive phase, 120, 121,
    122

Mineralocorticoids and immune
    reactions, 141, 151, 166, 170
  opposing effects to
    glucocorticoids, 166

Narcotic drugs, 6
  anaphylactic shock, 6
  inhibition of immune reactions, 6
  intensity of antibody formation,
    6

phagocytic reaction, 10
reticuloendothelial system, 6
Nervism, theory of, vii
Nervous activity, higher types of, 7
and immune reactions, 7, 8
Nervous system and immune
process, 13
Neurogenic theory in biomedical
sciences, viii
Neuroimmunomodulation, ix
Neurosis, inhibition of immune
reactions, 7
Nociceptive stimuli and immune
reactions, 24

Ontogenesis and effects of
hormones on immune
reactions, 155
Orienting reflexes and intensity of
antibody formation, 77

Parasympathetic nervous system,
effects on immune reactions,
151
Peyer's patches and stem cells of
bone marrow, 13
Phenoxybenzamine and
immunoblocking effects, 171

Reticular formation of midbrain,
39, 54
immune reactions, 39
plasma protein ratios, 39
Reticuloendothelial system, 47
influences on by medial and
posterior hypothalamus, 47

Serotonin-reactive brain structures
hypophysis transection, 53
stimulation, inhibits immune
reaction, 53
Sex hormones and immune

reactions, 143–45
chorionic gonadotropins, 144
diethylstilbestrol, 144
estrogen, 144
prolactin, 144
Shwartzman phenomenon, 137
Shwartzman-Sanarelli phenomena,
32
Somatotropin and immune
reaction, 141, 145, 146, 147
in ontogenesis, 155
Soporific drugs, 6
activity of reticuloendothelial
system, 6
inhibition of immune reactions, 6
intensity of antibody formation,
6
phagocytic activity, 6
Stress and immune reactions, 31
Stressor effects on immune
reactions, 114, 115, 143
Strychnine, intensification of
immune reactions, 6
Superior cervical sympathetic
ganglia
effects on initial stage of
immunogenesis, 20
stimulation and immunity, 18
transection and immunity, 17, 18,
19, 20, 21
Sympathetic nervous system
allergic reactions, 16
anaphylactic shock, 16, 17, 24
antibody production, 24–26
effects on thymus, 26, 27
gangliectomy and
immunogenesis, 17, 18
immune reactions, 14, 15, 16, 25
migration of stem cells from bone
marrow, 26–27
migration of thymus-dependent
lymphocytes, 26–27

production of stem cells by bone marrow, 26–27
Systems analysis of neurohumoral regulation of immune homeostasis, 159–61, 163, 164

Thymus, effects on development of the hypophysis, 149
Thyroid gland hormones and immune reactions, 145, 147, 148

Thyrotropin and immune reactions, 141, 145
T-lymphocytes, 13
Transcortin and immune reactions, 124, 125, 126, 133
Tuber cinereum
    effects of stimulation on allergic reactions, 40
    lesions and inhibition of anaphylactic shock, 32

D1639534